Prais...

"No matter what our stories hold, *A Hard Silence* is a book with a universal message of love, and the courage every single one of us needs to navigate our way to personal, familial, and communal healing."

MICHAEL PATRICK MACDONALD, AUTHOR OF
ALL SOULS: A FAMILY STORY FROM SOUTHIE

"Those of us whose family members were contaminated by HIV/AIDS around the same time shared her feelings, the agony of family secrecy and the fear of stigmatization."

VIC PARSONS, AUTHOR OF *BAD BLOOD: THE UNSPEAKABLE TRUTH*

"Melanie Brooks is that rare writer who can delve as deeply into the world of ideas as she can the pitted terrain of the human heart."

ANDRE DUBUS III, AUTHOR OF *GONE SO LONG* AND *TOWNIE*

"Fills me with a sense of urgency, gratitude, and awe."

ABIGAIL THOMAS, AUTHOR OF *STILL LIFE: THE NEXT INTERESTING THING*

"This beautifully rendered memoir asks important questions about the complexities of loss and grief, the roots of stigma and shame, and the courage necessary to endure that resonate in this new and unfortunate age of social exclusion."

RICHARD BLANCO, AUTHOR OF *THE PRINCE OF LOS COCUYOS: A MIAMI CHILDHOOD*

"A vivid and thoughtful exploration of a daughter's grief for her father, and a family's unwanted place in history, *A Hard Silence* movingly depicts the long toll of stigma and the healing power of words."

ALEX MARZANO-LESNEVICH, AUTHOR OF *THE FACT OF A BODY: A MURDER & A MEMOIR*

"A profound and riveting journey through shame and grief, *A Hard Silence* is, quite simply, unforgettable."

MONICA WOOD, AUTHOR OF *WHEN WE WERE THE KENNEDYS*

"Melanie Brooks writes with both daring and restraint about learning the language of loss and breaking the silence she grew up in during the 1980s and 1990s HIV/AIDS crisis."

KYOKO MORI, AUTHOR OF *YARN: REMEMBERING THE WAY HOME*

"With a documentarian's focus and the emotional armor necessary for re-entering a closely held decade-long family secret, Melanie Brooks takes us to fresh air found past that suffocating veil. Exquisitely written with big bravery and big heart."

SUZANNE STREMPEK SHEA, AUTHOR OF *SONGS FROM A LEAD-LINED ROOM*

"Melanie Brooks delivers an indelible portrait of love and loss in this brave exploration of the grief that was her constant companion after the death of her beloved father from AIDS... a beacon for all those who grieve."

MARIANNE LEONE, AUTHOR OF *JESSE: A MOTHER'S STORY* AND *MA SPEAKS UP*

"The strength required of Brooks to endure the cruel fate of her father's illness could have been surpassed only by what she summoned to write in this superb, heartfelt memoir... I could not put it down."

JERALD WALKER, AUTHOR OF *STREET SHADOWS* AND *THE WORLD IN FLAMES*

"*A Hard Silence* stands as an indictment of attitudes that add shame to suffering, that make struggling families hide, consigning their stories to silence. With artistry and courage, Brooks has turned that silence into this restorative, revelatory, and beautiful book."

RICHARD HOFFMAN, AUTHOR OF *HALF THE HOUSE* AND *LOVE & FURY*

"This searing memoir is a testament to the complex truth that our entitlement to grief is about so much more than loss and pain. Grief, for Brooks, is an act of memory."

JAED COFFIN, AUTHOR OF *ROUGHHOUSE FRIDAY*

About the Author

Melanie Brooks's first book, *Writing Hard Stories: Celebrated Memoirists Who Shaped Art from Trauma*, was published by Beacon Press in 2017. She teaches professional writing at Northeastern University and creative nonfiction in the MFA program at Bay Path University in Massachusetts. She earned an MFA in Creative Nonfiction from the University of Southern Maine's Stonecoast program. Her work has appeared in *Psychology Today*, the *HuffPost*, *Yankee Magazine*, *The Washington Post*, *Ms. Magazine*, *Creative Nonfiction*, and other notable publications. Though her Canadian roots run deep, she lives in New Hampshire with her husband, two children (when they are home from university), and two Labs.

melaniebrooks.com

a hard
silence

Dear Aaron —

One daughter remaps
family, grief, and faith when
HIV/AIDS changes it all

*So excited for our event in
October!*

MELANIE BROOKS

xx Melanie

www.vineleavespress.com

Permission obtained for quotes from:

Lewis, C.S. A Grief Observed. United Kingdom: Faber and Faber, Ltd., 1961.

Paul Farmer and Arthur Kleinman, "AIDS as Human Suffering," Daedalus, 118:2, pp. 135-162. © 1989 by the American Academy of Arts and Sciences.

Messenger, Orville and Dorothy Messenger, Borrowed Time: A Surgeon's Struggle With Transfusion-Induced AIDS. Oakville: Mosaic Press, 1995.

"Heavy" by Mary Oliver Reprinted by the permission of The Charlotte Sheedy Literary Agency as agent for the author. Copyright © 2006 by Mary Oliver with permission of Bill Reichblum

Dylan Thomas. "Do Not Go Gentle Into That Good Night." Copyright by Dylan Thomas Trust.

Cover design by Jessica Bell
Interior design by Amie McCracken

For Dad

Author's Note

This book is an intimate glimpse into one life deeply affected by the AIDS epidemic of the 1980s. The tragedy that unfolded in my family is rooted in a rarely acknowledged piece of a larger cultural story. I can only speak to that larger story as one who lived on the periphery of the communities most impacted by this illness, so I have not attempted to provide a comprehensive history of the AIDS crisis in these pages. That history already exists in powerful journalistic and personal accounts that describe what it was like for members of the LGBTQ+ community to face, en masse, the discrimination and stigma entrenched in this disease and to grieve the catastrophe of so many lives cut short at unfathomable rates. With profound respect and compassion for that community, I tell my story because there was no space into which my family and I fit as we dealt with AIDS outside any recognized group. We lived our experience in isolation and secrecy, bearing the burden of my father's illness and the certainty of his impending death from behind a curtain of silence. In writing this book, I've drawn back that curtain and voiced the story I needed to tell. That story is told from memory, so my recollections of events, conversations, and settings may be flawed, as memory tends to be. In some cases, I have altered people's names to protect their privacy. The way we talk about HIV/AIDS has changed since the onset of the epidemic. Overall, I have tried to avoid stigmatizing language, but at times I have used terminology representative of the era. In reflecting on this narrative against the backdrop of COVID-19, I see an ongoing chance for us to do better for those who have suffered the greatest Coronavirus losses. Physical distance defined this latest pandemic, but emotional distance need not. My fervent hope is that *A Hard Silence* might show those who are unable or not allowed to do so in the most difficult circumstances that they, too, can begin to speak the truths of their experiences and perhaps find they aren't so alone after all.

Prologue

A LITTLE OVER a year before his own, my father attends a funeral. It's Saturday, September 17, 1994. Somewhere inside the expansive Cathedral Church of All Saints in the South End of Halifax, Nova Scotia, he sits, deliberately beyond the reach of any camera lens there to capture the sea of recognizable faces of the over 600 mourners—including local and national community leaders, news reporters, and a handful of provincial politicians. Tension rides the lines of his body as he hunches low in the wooden pew and grips my mom's hand for support. He wears his dark tailored suit, crisp white shirt, and satin tie, handsome and robust despite concerted efforts to make himself small. No visible physical signs yet forecast that in fifteen months, when his lungs are ravaged by pneumocystis pneumonia (PCP) and his body emaciated by other unidentified opportunistic infections, he will die.

White-robed choir members and participating officiants with red ribbons pinned at their hearts process down the long aisle of the narrow sanctuary to the front chancel, and the resonant timbre of the church's pipe organ fills the space with the rich notes of the Anglican hymn, "Alleluia! Sing to Jesus." Beneath the gothic architecture—ornate wood carvings, towering arches, and vaulted ceilings—the wooden pews and additional blue folding chairs are packed with the family, friends, and followers of thirty-eight-year-old Randy Conners. In the front row, Randy's widow, Janet, dressed in a long black gold-buttoned jacket over simple black slacks, leans her slim frame against her fourteen-year-old son as she dabs her tear-filled eyes with the tissue she clutches in her fist.

Four days earlier, Randy died from complications related to AIDS after a period of prolonged illness. In the final two years of his life, Randy's had become one of the most recognizable faces of a national tragedy: Canada's tainted blood scandal. Between 1980 and 1985, close to two thousand Canadians, most from within the hemophiliac community, were infected with HIV from contaminated blood. More than seven hundred have since died. A person with severe hemophilia, Conners had contracted HIV sometime in the early 1980s from Factor 8, a government approved blood-clotting product derived from donated human blood plasma. He'd learned of his infection in 1987. Despite Randy's doctors' repeated assurances that there was little chance he could infect his wife, the couple learned in 1989 that Janet was also HIV-positive.

The Conners's heartbreak encapsulates what has been characterized as Canada's "worst-ever" public health disaster. Despite mounting evidence that infected blood products were known to be transmitting HIV, administrators of Canada's blood supply were slow to implement adequate measures to protect the public. Appalling mismanagement by the Canadian Red Cross and its regulators and systemic corporate greed by blood-product manufacturers and distributors showed blatant disregard for public safety and allowed infected blood to be knowingly distributed nationwide. The tragedy is the result of a complicated web of action and inaction by the parties involved, whose biggest failures included a lack of proper screening to eliminate high risk donors, unnecessary delays in implementing available screening methods of the blood products for HIV, and fateful decisions to save money by using up inventory of suspected contaminated products.

By going public when stigma and discrimination toward people infected with HIV and people dying of AIDS-related illnesses dominated the cultural landscape, Randy and Janet Conners helped spark an investigation into the national blood system and campaigned for appropriate compensation for victims and their families. Their courage to come forward, stand in the open, and say, "This is what happened to us" made them sympathetic symbols and drew the nation's attention to this important piece of the larger AIDS story. The portrait of this singular family facing the calamity of this widely misunderstood disease broadened the scope of the public's beliefs about HIV/AIDS and the people it infected.

"Many of us simply live our lives. A few of us manage to do things that make a real difference in the lives of others. Randy Conners is one of those." The white-haired officiating minister's words reverberate throughout the cathedral and cue a poignant celebration of Conners's passion in life and his courage at death. A procession of speakers hails him a hero. "He wouldn't die until the job was done, no matter how much pain he was experiencing," Randy's best friend declares, his hand gripping the microphone, his voice deep and controlled. "He lived his whole life that way. He wouldn't quit until the job was done."

Even while his health failed, Randy Conners lobbied until Nova Scotia became the first of Canada's provinces to award a comprehensive compensation package to victims of the tainted blood scandal—ensuring ongoing care and support for their families.

Mine was one of those families.

In contrast to Randy and Janet Conners's public crusade, my father and mother lived in the shadows for nine years after my father contracted HIV from a blood transfusion during open-heart surgery in 1985. They remained separated from the public narrative of the scandal, protecting our family's privacy and building a shield around my father's illness. Fear of its stigma, particularly within their evangelical Christian community where vocal condemnation of people infected with HIV and their "sinful lifestyles" was the norm, prompted that silence.

Twenty-five years later, I peer into this moment on the timeline of my family history, imagining and reimagining the scene, probing why my father braved that space and risked recognition despite his fear of exposure.

"They had a similar experience. I think he just felt like he wanted to pay his respects," my mother says when I pose the question on a recent visit home. The years that stretch beyond have muted her memory of that day, and, unlike me, she has little desire to pull shards of the past into the present landscape. For her this answer is enough. For me, it feels too obvious. Of course my father felt a kinship with this stranger. They'd lived less than ten miles apart, and Dad would have followed the news stories of Conners's struggles. Each had suffered similar bouts of debilitating illness. Each had feared for the future of their families. My father was one of the beneficiaries of the Nova Scotia compensation package Randy Conners fought for in the last years of his life.

Maybe Dad's presence speaks to his own longing to have this display of solidarity—these compassionate words of support, spoken openly in a house of worship—served to him. Is he quietly staging his own dress rehearsal? Is he testing himself to see if he can stand this close to the truth of his disease and remain intact? To see the people close by who will lean in to the tragedy of this illness? Does he need to hear the words "injustice" and "victim" spoken aloud to claim them for himself?

Like so many other daughters thinking about their fathers, as a little girl, I believed mine invincible. Nothing could alter the all-powerful, all-knowing largeness of who he was. And to my enamored mind, this picture was exactly as it should be. Only now, imagining him in that Halifax cathedral in 1994, longing to understand him in that moment, do I consider the possibility that he, too, had once embraced the same belief in himself. He was a surgeon, after all, and even though humility and compassion were the cornerstones of his practice, he must have internalized some of the god complex mentality that permeates the surgical culture. How else could he have rallied the courage to step into the operating room day after day to literally hold someone else's life in his hands? Over time, as my certainty of his invincibility shattered, I knew that the loss of his career, the worsening physical effects of one infection after another, and the daily dread of what lay ahead left him in turmoil. I watched him shrink beneath the weight of this disease, but until I imagined him facing his death, I didn't recognize the cruelty of his long season of waiting: the erasure of the invincible self he once carried at his core.

Maybe my father's need to bear witness to Randy Conners's funeral was less about what had happened to Randy Conners and more about what was still happening to him. Did participating in that community of grief, however clandestinely, feel like a chance to retrace the contours of his life and claim his place in this story?

Did he wonder then, as I do now, what it might have been like if we had, like the Conners, been part of the public battle sooner? What kind of support would have surrounded our suffering? Would my family's community of faith have responded, like this one, with a compassion that might have eclipsed shame?

I can forever spin these questions, but the truth is, their answers are beyond my reach. They inhabit the hard silence that defined my life and my family for nine lonely years. A silence I was made to carry throughout my adolescence and into my early adulthood. A silence I took with me when only two months before Randy Conners's death, I left home newly married and about to launch my own life a thousand miles away. A thousand miles from where my parents verged on unburdening themselves from their secret and stepping into the relief of being known.

Lost somewhere in that distance and physical separation is the permission I believed I needed to break free, too—the new set of family rules that would help me navigate a world where the secret was no longer necessary. My silence lingered for almost twenty more years and created a barrier that hid from view the complicated layers of my story. Only in peeling back those layers do I understand that the only permission I need to speak is my own.

MAPPING GRIEF

I thought I could describe a state; make a map of sorrow.
Sorrow, however, turns out to be not a state but a process.
It needs not a map, but a history...

C.S. LEWIS,
A Grief Observed

Heart Aches
1996

"HERE'S WHAT YOU need to do," my mom began, the cadence of her voice evoking calm. "Take a deep breath and put it out of your head for now so you can focus on your students and what they need from you today."

It was January, and my husband, Chris, and I had just returned to our home in Baltimore. I'd gone back to teaching social studies at a private Catholic girls' high school. In the preceding three weeks, we'd been in Halifax, Nova Scotia, sitting at Dad's bedside as he took his last breaths, then memorializing his life with family and friends, burying him on a frigid December day in a small, country cemetery, and enduring the first lonesome Christmas without him.

That morning, I sat at my classroom desk scanning lesson plans in the quiet interval between my early arrival and my students' entrance. The hovering pain of my loss butted against the looming responsibilities of my teaching day, and the terrible load of it all undid me. The stillness of the morning felt suddenly suffocating. My heart pounded in my chest so loudly that I could hear it in my ears, and my breath caught in my throat. I grabbed my cell phone, punched in my mother's phone number and whispered between heaving sobs that I didn't think I could survive the next minute, let alone the entire day.

"You need to stop thinking about it. Just breathe." I followed her instructions and forced my attention away from the sadness and back to my teaching notes. The air returned to my lungs, and my heartbeat slowed. "You'll be okay. You can do this, Melanie," Mom said.

"I can do this," I repeated and hung up the phone.

In the following days, I had a few more of these episodes, but this new strategy of disconnecting from the grief, quarantining it, enabled me to manage my classes and function, and the panic eventually subsided. It didn't occur to me to question why the panic happened. Until, that is, the day almost twenty years later, when it came back.

—

I pushed through the revolving hospital door and drew a ragged breath. The cold winter air filled my lungs on this day in 2011. My boots splashed through slushy pools as I speed-walked across the crowded parking lot, desperate for the solitude of my Trailblazer. With trembling hands, I jammed the keys into the ignition and started the engine. A frigid blast from the heater vent blew into my face, and I hit the button on the dash to slow the flow of air until it warmed up. Clutching the steering wheel with my gloved hands, I stared out the front windshield. The other parked cars melted into a clouded puddle behind my tears. The tightening vice in my chest squeezed, making it impossible to breathe. I needed to escape, but I couldn't move.

Words of reprimand tumbled through my brain: *This is ridiculous. They just said you are okay. What the hell is wrong with you?*

I closed my eyes and leaned back against the headrest. I focused on relaxing my muscles, trying to release the tension that gripped my entire body. I managed to gasp in a single breath before a cataclysm of sobs two decades in the making tore up my throat.

I was not okay.

Less than an hour before my disintegration into a mess of panic and immobilization, my heart had appeared on the flat-screen of a video monitor. In the dim light of a small hospital exam room, I'd watched its rhythmic motion as the sonographer isolated various views of ventricles and chambers, moving the ultrasound wand beneath my breast.

"Breathe normally," she'd instructed. This was the first time since I'd arrived that I'd heard her talk. Her words made me realize I was holding my breath. I released the air in a slow stream.

She clicked a few more images and pointed out the different chambers of my heart and then the septum, the muscle partition between the right and left ventricles. "This is what we watch during the stress echo," she said. "If there's a blockage, we'll see a difference in the way this muscle moves."

I swallowed hard and clenched the sides of the exam table. A bloom of heat rushed through my body despite the icy ultrasound gel. Even though I couldn't actually feel the sensation, I was watching *my* heart pulse away on the monitor. This was *my* blood circulating. These were *my* muscles pumping. And I was not in control of any of it.

When I was pregnant with my son, Will, I had my first ultrasound at the eighteen-week mark. I had started to feel small, sporadic flutters of movement tickling me from the inside. When the screen filled with the undeniable shape of a baby moving and kicking and rolling, I'd had a hard time bridging the mental gap that connected him to me. He had the hiccups, and his little body convulsed every two to three seconds. But I felt nothing. Mingling with my excitement in that moment, an urgent desire crept in to stop time so I could decipher the puzzle.

Seeing my heart pumping on the monitor this time, I had the same reaction.

"Are you feeling any chest pain today?" Becky, the nurse on the other side of the table, asked. She was the one running the show here. I couldn't take my eyes off her bouncing hair every time I looked at her. Tightly rolled, Shirley Temple curls covered her head, each one shaped by either a hot iron or roller. It seemed like she'd missed a step in the coiffing process, though, and forgotten to comb through the ringlets to create a finished style. Instead, she had the appearance of having left the beauty parlor in a rush halfway through her appointment. She was one of those non-stop talkers, overly chipper and too eager to put me at ease.

It didn't work.

"No pain today," I said.

But in the weeks earlier, there had been. An occasional tightness in my upper left side and increasing numbness in my left arm prompted my doctor to order this test. "Just to rule out any problems," he promised, his demeanor indicating he wasn't worried. I trusted him then, but, in this moment, with electrodes stuck to my chest beneath a flimsy gown and twisted lead wires connecting to a computer charged with determining the fitness of my heart, I began to doubt.

Becky guided me from the exam table to the treadmill against the wall and started it up. She explained the procedure. Every three minutes, the speed and incline of the treadmill would increase incrementally with the goal of increasing my heart rate as well. "This test can be tough. Most people average about six to eight minutes before stopping." She'd just laid down the gauntlet.

Well, damn, Crazy Curls, I thought as the belt beneath my sneakered feet began to move. I'm a runner. I run four or five miles at least three times a week. I can last longer than the "average" six to eight minutes. Bring it on. I'll show you a healthy heart. Watching the numbers on Becky's screen, my confidence solidified. I could see the targeted heart rate and mine remained well below the line for the first interval. After three minutes the treadmill sped up and the incline steepened. It was still totally doable and didn't require much more effort.

Becky wanted me talking as the test progressed, and she found the perfect topic. She'd recognized my last name and realized that she knew my in-laws. "I used to go to youth group at Trinity Baptist with your father-in-law when we were teenagers!" she exclaimed as she typed something into the computer and the next three-minute interval began.

Great, I thought and focused my eyes on a chip in the yellow paint on the wall in front of me. My husband's family had a long history in our town in New Hampshire that went back two generations. It was not uncommon to run into people who knew his parents. A lot of those connections hearkened back to their evangelical roots and involvement in the Baptist church that Chris's grandfather helped found. I shared similar roots, but I'd been distancing myself from them lately. That, and the fact that my in-laws could run hot and cold in their relationships and often lost connection to people always made these encounters feel awkward and uncertain, like I owed the recipient some sort of excuse.

My temples thrummed. Without looking at the screen, I knew my heart rate was climbing. My breathing grew labored, and it was getting harder to answer Crazy Curls's questions about what my mother-in-law and father-in-law had been up to in the last forty years. At nine minutes, the speed and incline shifted again, and my heart rate leapt into the targeted zone as beads of perspiration formed on my forehead. I could no longer speak, and my breaths came in quick, uncontrolled gasps. I jogged, but with the steep slant, it felt like running full tilt up a hill. At twelve minutes, I called it quits.

"That was great!" Becky chirped and helped me off the treadmill. I lay back down on the exam table. The paper covering crinkled underneath me. My pulse pounded as the sonographer, who I now understood was the silent, unnamed sidekick to counter Becky's chatter, captured the requisite images. This time, I had no trouble connecting the pumping heart on the screen to the intense beating in my chest. This final testing phase called for me to lie still and stay quiet.

As I did, my eyes followed the rotating blades of the ceiling fan over-head, and in those muted seconds, a surge of apprehension climbed my spine. The muscles in my torso locked. A taste like sucking silver was on my tongue. Already winded from the exertion of the treadmill, I struggled to draw in enough air.

My head was immersed in a sea of questions and images. What did these two women see on that screen that I might not? What if there *was* something wrong with my heart? The possibility was not remote. My dad's beloved face—his eyes shining behind his wire-rimmed glasses, his cheeks creasing into long dimples with his characteristic smile—flashed in my mind. I'd watched his trajectory of "early onset cardiac issues," the words my primary care physician used when he'd prescribed this test, play out at extremely close range. I'd watched the unforeseen consequences of those issues and his subsequent heart surgery dismantle the life he'd created for himself and our family. I didn't want to travel any part of that path again. And I didn't want any fragments of that pain for my children or husband, either. Thoughts of Will and Lily dealing with a sick mother, or of Chris carrying worry, made me almost cry out.

Becky finally spoke and her words suspended my anxious spiral. "The cardiologist will take a quick look," she said, "but everything looks really good." I willed my breathing to return to normal and pulled myself into a sitting position. I dropped my legs over the side of the table and reached for my t-shirt and bra on the chair in the corner as Becky turned to follow the sonographer out of the room so I could get dressed.

Before she left, she turned back and said, "You're only forty, right? That's young to be having a stress test. Is there a history of heart disease in your family?"

"My father had a heart attack at forty-two."

"Did he survive?"

I hesitated then, and the question hung unanswered between us for a beat too long. The real answer, a grenade of turbulent emotion that would detonate in a few minutes when I left the hospital and reached my car, could not be explained in this limited space of time.

"Yes," I said finally, and a different kind of ache intensified in my heart—one that couldn't be measured by electrodes and sophisticated monitors. "He survived."

It's Complicated
2011

THE DAY I started releasing my quarantine grief, I didn't think to wear waterproof mascara. That morning, when I'd leaned close to my bathroom mirror and gone through my routine of brushing the makeup onto my lashes, the thought that I might want the other option, the one with "staying power" hadn't crossed my mind. In my defense, I didn't know that I was going to be releasing any of my grief that day. Crying was the last thing I planned when I walked into the therapist's office for my first session, my back straight, my head held high. Composure was my superpower. I rarely broke down, and if I did, I didn't do it in front of other people. Especially people who were strangers.

Yet, ten minutes in, I was a disaster. My breath hiccupped from my mouth in choked gasps. Streams of black undoubtedly created murky rivers down my cheeks; snot dripped. I called on every reserve of will-power to stay seated instead of jumping up and fleeing. A Kleenex box taunted me from a table at the opposite end of the leather couch. Hard as I tried, I couldn't figure out a discreet way to reach for it.

The therapist sat across from me in a high-backed upholstered chair, his fingers laced loosely over his knees. His gaze was steady. He appeared unfazed by my dramatic dissolution into this heap of incoherence. Sunlight streamed in through the window over his shoulder. On this December day, a brilliant blue sky framed the leafless trees and tall evergreens rising from the cemetery across the street.

"I don't usually do this," I managed to stutter on the tail end of a sob, motioning toward my face. I couldn't meet his gaze.

"It's not unusual," Dr. B said, his tone calm. Caring. I guessed he was in his mid-to-late fifties. With his thin, graying hair, neatly trimmed goatee, earth-toned tweed jacket over a blue button-down dress shirt, this guy fit perfectly with the shrink image I'd formulated. Add a pipe in his hand and a golden retriever at his feet, and he could be an icon from a Norman Rockwell painting. "There's a lot of anxiety and uncertainty at play when people choose to try counseling," he said. "I see this a lot."

I tried to decide if his words were reassuring or not. It was encouraging to know I was not a freak, but something about his statement challenged the originality of my experience. The last thing I wanted to be was a cliché. How many people like me, teetering on the edge of midlife and in search of solid ground to stand on, did this guy see?

A low bookshelf against the wall to my left was filled with titles like: *Helping Children Manage Their Anger, The Denial of Death, The Steady Heart, The Anger Trap, ADD/ADHD and Other Behavioral Disorders, Managing Your Anxiety and Worry, Overcoming Sexual Addiction.* That one gave me pause, and, for a moment, I wondered about the other people that visited this office. A green trench coat and a leather driving hat hung from a hook on the door. His desk was crowded with stacks of manila folders, a laptop, telephone, and trays of papers. A five-drawer, metal file cabinet fit neatly in the corner. Three framed diplomas were on display behind his desk. The middle one was crooked.

I'd had a plan when I got there. A plan to solve a specific problem. My new panic problem. A panic that followed me around everywhere and latched onto everything, leaving me feeling like I was losing my footing. And—especially when I was sitting in my car, hyperventilating and frozen—like I was losing my mind. "A little stress resulting from some recent changes in my life," I said when I called to make this appointment.

I might have underplayed things a bit.

What I dubbed my "psychological freefall" started with a rejection letter two months earlier from a Master of Fine Arts program to which I'd applied—a program I'd hoped would be a salve for an inexplicable restlessness in my mind and body and be the excuse I needed to write. A program that might let me escape the drudgery I was feeling in my teaching life as a part-time college writing instructor. I didn't plan on rejection. And I didn't plan on the deep disappointment that trailed it.

Then, a month before that first appointment, Chris and I walked away from church. Just like that. We uprooted ourselves and our two children from a lifetime investment in the evangelical Christian community because we couldn't gel our thinking with its thinking. Our church congregation was becoming vocal in its conservative leanings, specifically in its lack of acceptance toward the LGBTQ+ community. My brother David is gay, and when we recognized that he and my brother-in-law, Ian, would never be welcome in our church, and that well-meaning Sunday school leaders might teach our children that they were supposed to feel something other than love for their uncles, we knew we had to leave. I wasn't sure if I ever wanted to go back to church again.

This uncertainty was rocking my confidence. And that, along with the inconvenient episodes of chest pain that resulted in uneasy conversations with cardiac nurses, was making me panic. When I panicked, I felt out of control. I needed to be in control. So, emboldened by the recent discovery that one of my best friends was also seeing this therapist, I set up an appointment to solve the problem.

Clearly, things weren't going according to plan.

"I really don't do this," I said again to Dr. B, and this time I faced him, trying to read him.

His eyes were crystal blue, a tint of ocean on a cloudless day, and so, so kind. The kind eyes, coupled with his gentle "So how are you doing?" not long after I sat down, were what undid me. That was all it took. I replayed the earlier portion of my day: walking Lily to school, running in and out of the grocery store to grab a few staples, stopping for gas, picking up the dry cleaning, and mailing a couple of boxes of Christmas presents to my nieces and nephews in Canada. A lot of people had asked me how I was doing. Not once did the question make me wish I'd worn waterproof mascara.

But there, in that space that was meant for honesty, when this kind-eyed stranger asked, I felt like he really wanted to know. I felt like maybe I could tell him. Except I didn't know how. I'd never tried therapy, and I'd never been offered this kind of open-ended invitation to speak.

"Not so great," I began, and something let go. Something let go and spilled everywhere.

The old grief was surfacing, and I had no clue what to do about it. How was I supposed to begin to explain the tears and the complicated history where they lived? How was I supposed to gracefully reach for a Kleenex? What made me ever believe this was a good idea?

The Beginning
1985

DAVID AND I climbed off the school bus and raced down our winding driveway, our coats unzipped to the warmth of the afternoon sun. Spring was in the air on this April day of my seventh-grade year. The tall pines that curtained most of our house from the road reached toward a cloudless sky. Mounds of dirty snow, the last remnants of winter, dotted the path to the house. We playfully shoved each other as we clambered up the steps of the side deck, each trying to be the first inside. Stomping into the house, we dropped our jackets, boots, and bags in heaps on the tiled floor of the back hallway and made a beeline to the kitchen to scavenge for snacks.

"Guys, can you come to my room for a minute?" Mom stood by the counter. The edge to her voice caught my attention, and I turned to look at her. Her face was the color of bone. Her red-rimmed eyes seemed abnormally bright. Her lips pressed into a thin, straight line.

Without speaking, Dave and I followed her down the carpeted hallway to her bedroom. She motioned for us to sit on her bed, and as I settled into the softness of the mattress, I noticed with alarm the laundry basket overflowing with unfolded clean clothes in the middle of the floor. Mom never left a task half-finished. Ever.

She spoke. "After Dad went to work today, he started feeling a lot of pain in his chest. The other doctors ran some tests, and they think he had a heart attack." Her words were quiet, but they screamed through my head. *Dad. Heart attack. It's Dad.* I was paralyzed. Tears sprang to my eyes and washed down my cheeks. A silent, repeating prayer began: Please God. Please. Make him be okay.

"Is Dad going to die?" David asked what I couldn't, his eyes wide, a tremor in his voice.

Mom looked at me over his head, her uncertainty dangling in the pause before her answer. She gave him a weak smile and took his hand. "No, Davey. He's at the hospital, and we're going to pick up Michael and Mark to go see him now. He's going to be okay." She reached for my hand, too, and before her fingers tightened to squeeze it, I felt them shaking.

We drove the fifteen minutes to my older brothers' high school without speaking, except for occasional questions from David as his logical mind tried to piece together the events. "What does a heart attack look like?" "Did Daddy faint?" "Is he in bed?" "Who is taking care of his patients?" "Who is looking after him?" I stared out the passenger window. We passed by my friend Rhonda's long driveway, and I remembered my promise on the bus to bike over after I finished my homework. Would she be mad when I didn't show up? The wide fields and dense trees of Gorge Road thinned as we crossed the Trans-Canada and turned onto Mountain Road toward the center of Moncton, New Brunswick, where cookie-cutter houses crowded into subdivisions. We passed Deluxe Fish & Chips, a favorite take-out restaurant. I didn't feel comforted by the familiar landscape of my hometown whizzing by. Even though I knew this route by heart, I felt lost.

We pulled up next to Moncton High School. With its stone walls, arched wooden doors and central tower, it looked more like a Gothic castle than a school. It was the same high school where my parents met when they were fourteen years old. The day's final classes were dismissing. A crowd of teenagers streamed out the entrance into the parking lot.

Mom got out and stood in front of the car to make sure my brothers saw her. Backpacks slung over their shoulders, Michael and Mark greeted my mother with broad smiles, delighted that they would not be subject to the long bus ride home. Their smiles vanished as soon as she began to speak, and, as they climbed into the car, I watched their faces contort with the same confusion and fear that must have been stamped on mine.

It was a quick ride from the high school to the Moncton Hospital. The red brick of the building came into view when we turned onto Macbeath Avenue. I knew this place. My dad, a general and thoracic surgeon, was the chief of surgery there. This was his "office," though he did have an actual one in another building a few blocks away. On the frequent nights when his dinner sat cold on the table, and Mom gave us permission to go ahead with ours without his presence, I would imagine him behind these walls. I'd picture him walking down the hallway, his shoulders hunched slightly from the boyhood years he toted a heavy newspaper bag across his chest to deliver to the neighborhoods of this town. He'd be dressed in green scrubs, a stethoscope hanging around his neck, his head bent over the chart of a sick patient who, in that moment when the food on Dad's plate went untouched, needed him more than we did.

We made our way through the winding corridors following the signs and arrows leading us to cardiology. There had been a few occasions when I'd trailed Dad in these same halls, times when Mom brought me and the boys to see him for a quick visit when shifts on call kept him there overnight. On those days, I'd loved the current of energy that hummed in the hospital air. People were always moving. Nurses pushed gowned patients in wheelchairs, IV bags rolling behind on tall, stainless-steel rods. Uniformed orderlies traveled in and out of doorways with stacks of white linens or carts lined with trays of food. A chorus of buzzers and alarms and phones and pagers sang around us. And doctors like my dad walked while scrutinizing shadowy X-rays raised to the fluorescent ceiling lights or reading through patient histories on clipboard charts.

This time, without Dad as guide, the hospital's activity scared me. The light seemed too bright, and the urgent movement of those same nurses, orderlies, and doctors, unsettling. The disinfectant smell made me dizzy. I couldn't look away from patients we passed, their skin gray and their bodies folded as they shrunk into wheelchairs. I now under-stood the expression I saw on each of their faces. They were scared too.

After the nurse at the desk told us that Dad had gone for more tests, Mom ushered us into a tiny waiting room off the hallway of the cardi-ology wing. There were just enough plastic chairs for the five of us. Outdated magazines lay scattered on a couple of faux-wood tables, and a lamp in the corner cast a dingy glow around the room. My brothers and I sat quiet and unsure, lost in imagining what might be coming.

Without warning, Mom reached for the trashcan in the corner, lifted it to her face, and vomited. Michael, sixteen, the dutiful oldest child, rubbed her back and spoke soothing words. She leaned into him for support. I was the only girl, stuck in the middle, uncertain what role I played in this moment when everything was wrong. I had nowhere to lean, so I curled into myself, squeezing my fear like a fist. My prayer changed. Please God. Let us *all* be okay.

After ten minutes, a different nurse led us to Dad's room. She was dressed in a pink uniform, a white name badge that I couldn't read hanging from her pocket. Her ponytail swung in a distracting rhythm. Mom disappeared through the doorway first, recovered and overly cheerful, and we filed behind, falling into our birth order: Michael, Mark, then me, and, finally, David. As the others surrounded the bed, I held back, my breath stuck in my throat, unable to get my legs to carry me forward to where Dad, my invincible dad, was lying in a hospital bed. His eyes were sunken and tired, his face pale. An oxygen mask covered his mouth, fogging with each strained breath. Wires twisted from beneath his thin gown, somehow connecting him to the beeps and squiggly lines tracing their way across the monitor beside his bed. From a half-filled bag of dripping fluid, a long, clear tube snaked down to a taped needle puncturing the top of his hand. An ugly, purple bruise eclipsed the remaining visible skin.

I wanted to tell him to get up. Scream, "Get up and be you! This isn't you! You are strong. You are the doctor, not the patient. You are Dad. Get up. Be Dad. Please." Instead, I bit my lip, holding back the sob that threatened to escape.

"Hi Meligans," he said to me, moving the mask away from his face with his untethered hand. He smiled his dad smile. His cheeks creased into long dimples and his soft, brown eyes crinkled behind the square lenses of his glasses.

Still unsure of my voice, I stepped toward the bed and took his extended hand. His warm fingers closed over mine.

"I bet this isn't what you guys expected today," he tried to joke, a glimmer that he was still there behind the mask, the wires, the weakened body. He was still Dad working his dad humor to ease our worry. We crowded closer, all searching for a spot, grasping to hold on to this beloved man who anchored our family.

Dad would not remember any of this. Later that night, after test results determined the severity of his condition, he'd be taken by ambulance the three hours to the Victoria General Hospital in Halifax better equipped for cardiac patients. Doctors there would make a plan of action. After his eventual operation, there would be a permanent hole in Dad's immediate short-term memory—a common side effect for patients put on heart-lung machines during bypass surgery. The events of this day and the days that followed would come to him secondhand. Mom would shield him by leaving out painful details. She would use the words "quite upset" when she described our reactions to seeing him in this terrifying condition. She would not tell him of the agony that permeated the room, choking me with its grip, when we four children stood at Dad's bedside and put on brave smiles for him as he prepared for a journey to somewhere we didn't understand, somewhere from which he might not come back. She would not tell him how we each endured a wrenching moment of separating from him before we exited the room. She would not tell him about when I leaned in, kissed his cheek, and said, "I love you, Daddy" and watched him falter as tears collected in his eyes when he whispered back, "I love you, too, my Melanie Joybells." It was goodbye. Just in case.

She would not tell him, and he would not remember.

But I would. With the resonance of a movie watched over and over again, I would forever remember every detail from this scene.

I exited my Sunday school classroom with the other seventh graders and headed toward the church's fellowship hall to find my brothers and my aunt Joan, my mom's oldest sister. She'd flown in from Montreal to stay with us while Mom sat at Dad's bedside in Halifax, waiting for what came next. It had been almost a week since his heart attack.

I wandered into the open room where tables covered in paper table-cloths had been set with glasses of lemonade, Styrofoam cups filled with coffee, and plates of cookies—snacks for the interval between Sunday school and the worship service. The praise chorus we'd sung at the end of my class still hummed in my head as I scanned the crowd of familiar faces for my family. "Father, I adore you / Lay my life before you / How I love you."

For the last six days, a numbness had engulfed my body. I'd gone through the motions of daily living. I'd sat at my desk at school and recited memorized lines from Robert Frost's "Stopping by Woods on a Snowy Evening," solved geometry problems, and discussed Canada's Articles of Confederation. I'd gone to my friends' houses to hang out, dutifully practiced my flute, and swum laps at swimming lessons. I'd tried to ignore the widening divide I felt between my peers and me, a chasm that now separated us into two categories: kids who didn't have fathers who might be dying, and me, the girl with the father who quite possibly could be.

Today we were at First Baptist Church, praying alongside family friends for Dad's speedy recovery. God worked miracles. We could all point to the Bible verses that told us so. We knew the stories, and we believed them.

The heritage of Christian faith ran deep in my family. My father's father was a Baptist minister. His call to ministry took him from a tiny mining town in England's Lake District to Canada in the 1920s and then overseas as a chaplain in the Canadian Armed Forces during World War II.

My mother's father was the son of Christian missionaries, and he'd spent the first fifteen years of his life living in Northern China while his parents worked to spread the gospel to remote areas. A room was at the ready in my mother's childhood home for missionaries on furlough. Throughout her youth, people who'd sacrificed everything in the service of God surrounded her. My parents' childhood homes placed God at the center and dictated strict moral codes of behavior against the sinful trappings of the secular world. Before going to college, my father had never set foot in a movie theater.

Naturally, my parents' evangelical Christian roots wrapped around my brothers and me. Sunday school, weekly worship services, Bible studies, Christian fellowship events—all were at the center of my childhood and adolescence. The words of hymns and scripture were engraved on my brain. I grew up loving Jesus. That love was a part of my DNA. It never occurred to me that I had a choice. And, until the week of my father's heart attack, it never occurred to me that God wasn't listening to my faithful prayers.

I saw Michael and Mark walking toward me from the other side of the fellowship hall. There was a particular importance in Michael's stride that told me he carried news.

"Mom just called the church office," he said. "Dad's going to have open-heart surgery first thing tomorrow morning. We have to go to Halifax today. Now."

I gulped a mouthful of air and held it.

—

Different hospital. Different city. Same disinfectant smell.

And now, interminable waiting.

Despite being on the 11th floor, its large windows overlooking the expanse of Halifax's downtown, the sterile sameness of the waiting room's white walls stifled me. Michael and Mark read in the corner, both hunched low in their seats. We were the only people in this surgical waiting room, and we'd taken it over. I'd been trying to read, too, but Jessica and Elizabeth Wakefield, the twin heroines of *Sweet*

Valley High, kept repeating their dialogue as my eyes traveled across the same paragraph over and over. I couldn't sit still any longer. David, lying on his stomach on the floor, lined up his Matchbox cars according to color and size, but I could see from the way he was kicking his legs that he felt fidgety too. He was only eight. At thirteen, I could barely make sense of what was happening. He was so little. How could he?

"Mel, why don't you and David take a little walk down the hallway? Stretch your legs?" Mom suggested, looking up from her knitting, the needles continuing to move and create even without her scrutiny. A thread of cream-colored yarn wound up from the quilted floral bag on the floor to the sleeve of the cabled sweater she was working on. Worry was written into the lines on her forehead even though she tried to sound upbeat.

"Come on," I said, standing and motioning to David. "Maybe we can find a snack." His blue eyes lit up at the mention of food, and he shifted the line of cars to the side and stood too. We dug in Mom's wallet and found some quarters before we headed out the door and onto the main floor, our shoes slapping against the linoleum and echoing down the hallway. It was deserted and felt almost haunted. In this section of the hospital, most of the activity took place behind the tall steel doors we passed, labeled *AUTHORIZED PERSONNEL ONLY.*

Dad was behind one of those doors. This was the backdrop I saw when I pictured him at work. But this was not his hospital. This time, he was not the guy wearing the green scrubs and holding the scalpel, in charge and making the life-saving decisions.

He was the patient.

Somewhere, deep in the labyrinth of this surgical wing, he was lying on a table while another surgeon grafted vessels from his leg to the vessels of his heart so that the blood could flow through them. His chest was open, his ribs spread apart, his heart exposed, and his life rested in somebody else's hands.

Around the next corner, David and I found the sought-after snacks. A vending machine supplied us with M&Ms and Potato Stix.

"Do you want to split them?" I asked when we sat on a black bench next to the machine.

"Sure." David moved closer.

We divided our bounty, counting the M&Ms to make it an even trade. David, usually the chatterbox, stayed quiet as we ate, seeming to understand that I didn't want to talk. The mix of chocolate and salt on my tongue tasted good. Better than the stale, powdered donut I'd had for breakfast from the hotel where we'd spent the night.

"We should head back," I said when he popped the last M&M into his mouth.

He followed me down the corridor toward the waiting room. We rounded the corner, and one of the tall doors opened in our path. I grabbed David's arm, halting him mid-step. With our backs to the wall, we watched as a nurse in blue scrubs, a surgical mask covering her face, held the door open. Two other nurses, dressed the same way, grasped a gurney by its metal rails and wheeled it through the opening. Others walked with them, clutching machines and IV poles connecting to the patient on the bed. I tightened my hold on David's arm and my throat constricted.

The patient was Dad.

A shower cap covered his head and his face was partially obscured by a breathing tube taped to his mouth. Its other end attached to a machine wheeled by one of the nurses. Hissing air flowed through the tube mechanically filling and emptying his lungs. His eyes were closed. The exposed skin of his neck and chest was a rusty orange—iodine antiseptic brushed on to remove all traces of bacteria.

Dr. Murphy, Dad's cardiac surgeon, walked with the procession. His hand rested on the end of the moving bed in an authoritative and protective gesture. He wore a blue surgical cap and sweat darkened the fabric against his forehead. His mask hung wrinkled around his neck.

We'd met him that morning next to Dad's bedside before they'd wheeled him to surgery. It had been a relief to see Dad again after the long week of waiting, but soon after our arrival, we'd had to reenact an almost identical farewell scene to the last one. There had been less intensity this time, though. Since Dr. Murphy and Dad were both surgeons, there was an ease to their interaction. "Make the incisions straight," Dad joked. "I don't want crooked scars." Dr. Murphy laughed along with him, promising to account for all the clamps at the end too. The mood in the room had been light. Bearable.

Dr. Murphy turned with the gurney and noticed David and me standing in the hallway. He paused. A hundred years passed before he spoke, and in that time, I felt it all: the heaviness of the wait, the uncertainty of the future, the paralyzing terror of losing my dad. It all rested on the words Dr. Murphy was about to say. I searched his face, and internally begged him to say what I wanted to hear.

"Well, this is someone you know," he affirmed, bending his tall frame closer, and a gentle smile broke on his face. He tussled David's sandy hair, and then looked at me. "It's finished. Everything went well. We'll get him comfortable, and then you guys can come down to see him."

Air filled my lungs fully for the first time in a week. My fear gave way and relief tiptoed up my spine as my eyes followed the wheeling gurney around the corner. I reached for David's hand, and we rushed to the waiting room to tell everyone the happy news. We'd seen Dad. He was alive. Everything was going to be okay.

—

What I know now is that I breathed too soon. My skin prickles when I look back and realize that in the moment I was restacking the foundational blocks of our family, optimistically picturing things returning to normal, exhaling my fear and inhaling welcome relief, *it* was already there.

The virus had hijacked the cells of the transfused blood given to Dad to keep him alive during surgery. *It*s undetected, malevolent journey started through the vessels of his newly mended heart, circulating through his veins, taking up residence in his body. Planning. Manipulating. Was *it* watching thirteen-year-old me in that hospital hallway? Did *it* see me loosen my grip on David's arm and lean my body against the wall while Dr. Murphy spoke? Did *it* feel my blooming hope? Was *it* laughing?

Whatever else *it* was doing just then, I know this for certain: AIDS was coursing into our world.

SECRECY AND SHAME

The AIDS epidemic brought with it a significant amount of stigma. When the AIDS epidemic first hit [,] people were afraid, afraid of what it was, afraid of what it could possibly do to them, afraid of the unknown.

GWENDOLYN BARNHART,
"The Stigma of HIV/AIDS," *American Psychological Association*

It Wasn't Cancer

2013

ON A SEPTEMBER evening, I leaned against the door of my friend Carol's tan Jeep in the parking lot next to the soccer fields where our daughters practiced. We chatted through the open passenger window. The final rays of sun receded over the tall pines that lined the far end of the field where boys and girls of varying ages, clad in the navy-and-silver jerseys of the Nashua, New Hampshire Cobras soccer club, chased balls and ran drills. The earthy smell of fresh-cut grass wafted from the pitch. A chain-link fence contained the players and the balls to the grassy terrain. Deep woods walled in three sides of this grid of fields, and the parking lot edged the fourth.

I watched Lily race up the field toward the net, her blonde ponytail bouncing. She faked left and trapped the ball, then swerved past one of the older girls, broke away and took a shot on goal. The shot hit the post, but Ariel, her trainer, gave her a high five. Lily had made a valiant effort and her footwork was improving. She loved that her Under-10 team trained with the Under-13 girls during practice. The early evening air carried the chill of fall. I pulled on my zippered sweatshirt.

"How was the summer?" I asked Carol. I hadn't seen her since school ended in June. We'd known each other since Will and her daughter, Melissa, started kindergarten, and her son, Danny, and Lily began preschool. They'd continued to travel through school together, and it was mainly kid events that connected Carol and me: field trips, ski club, soccer games, concerts, school open houses.

"Okay," she responded. She turned to face me with a weak smile. She tucked her blonde-streaked hair behind her ear. Her eyes, lined in black pencil, spoke something different than her words. Sadness dulled her gaze. She looked away, but not before I saw the welling tears.

The previous August, Carol's husband, Dave, had died of pancreatic cancer. Chris and I had taken the kids to the wake. It was their first one. After forcing Lily into a skirt and squeezing her feet into a too-small pair of ballet flats and making Will put on a collared shirt and his "nice" shorts (the ones with no stains) we'd taken a few minutes to talk things through. We explained the difference between a wake and a funeral. We prepared them for the possibility of an open casket and reassured them that they didn't have to go close to it if they didn't want to. Lily had widened her hazel eyes. Her mind registered the image, and her face contorted in a mixture of horror and disdain. "That's kind of gross!" she said finally.

"It really won't be gross," I said. "It will sort of look like Mr. Lavoie is sleeping." As the words left my mouth, I remembered reading somewhere that it was bad to compare death to sleep when talking to children. Something about them thinking they could die or someone they loved could die every time they went to sleep. I had to believe that Lily's logic was more grounded than that.

"What exactly are we supposed to do?" Lily had asked then. She needed to be prepared. Guidelines for what to expect secured her. She was like me that way.

"You just show up," I said. "You show up, and you tell Melissa and Danny that you're sad about their dad. It's how you give them support."

Will leaned against the butcher-block island in our kitchen looking down at his hands. He hadn't said anything, but I knew he was listening. He processed things quietly—a mini version of Chris.

"We won't stay a long time," Chris said. "They'll have a lot of family there, and other friends." Chris was not a lingerer. He was about getting the task done. He was also super sensitive to protocol in these circumstances because he'd worked for a funeral home in between undergrad and graduate school the year before we got married. Since we didn't fall into the category of family or close friends, we should not be milling around. I also knew he didn't want to subject the kids for longer than we needed to.

Or me, for that matter.

We walked up the steps toward the brick-lined entrance of the funeral home and my own unease was all I felt. I really hated wakes. I'd chosen not to mention this fact to the kids in our pep talk back at the house because it seemed counterproductive and hypocritical. Now, though, my flight instinct was poised to kick in. This is not about you, I kept repeating in my head.

It was, though. It always was.

When death became a part of my story, it somehow tangled me up with everyone's death stories. The ache of grief that settled in my bones when my father died intensified whenever I was face-to-face with someone else's loss.

A few men in dark suits stood by the door. One leaned over the railing taking long drags on a cigarette. He'd removed his jacket and slung it over the metal bar. Something in his face looked familiar, and I wondered if he might be one of Dave's brothers. I gave him a small smile and a quiet "Hello" as we herded the kids through the double doorway.

We stepped into a sunny foyer and felt the contrast of the air-conditioner to the summer heat outside. The walls were painted a soft yellow, trimmed with white. A cardboard placard with *David J. Lavoie* printed on it pointed us toward the corridor that led left. A wide entryway opened into the visitation room. Lily smashed her body into my side as we approached. Will walked next to Chris, his hands in his pockets. A registry book sat open on a small table, and I paused to sign our names before we entered. I glanced at Chris. "In and out," he said under his breath. I nodded.

We passed through the entryway, and I scanned the room to get my bearings. It wasn't crowded. We'd decided to come on the early side of the calling hours, hoping to avoid the mid-evening rush. A low buzz filled the space from the small groups of chatting visitors clustered in the center. I knew some faces: the PTO president and the principal from the elementary school stood talking to Danny's teacher for the upcoming year. High-backed chairs lined the wall, and some of the elderly family members had taken up positions there. The decor included bright bouquets of flowers varying in size and style, artfully arranged around the room.

The formal receiving line was to my left, and I glimpsed Carol wearing a simple black dress standing next to a line of people I assumed were relatives. She was engaged in a conversation with a middle-aged couple whose backs were to us. The casket was beside her. It was open, but I didn't look long enough to register the details. I needed to ease my way over.

I focused instead on the large posters of family photos that were propped up on easels. Dave's life captured in snapshots of pivotal moments: family vacations, holidays, school events, and activities. Melissa was standing to the left of the entryway near one of the easels. Flanked by two other girls I recognized from Will's grade, she giggled and talked with them in whispers. When they caught sight of Will, they hurried over and dragged him away from the easel. "Don't you dare look at the baby pictures!" Melissa warned, the pitch of her voice rising with each word. Will followed them to the side of the room, his hands still stuffed in his pockets.

Chris and I walked Lily to where Danny was standing with another boy from their class. Smart of Carol to give the kids allies for these moments. Relief for them and for her, I imagined. Danny wore a white dress shirt with the sleeves rolled to his elbows, and a striped tie. Unlike Melissa, he was all business. "Thanks for coming," he said to Lily.

"You're welcome," she replied and stepped easily into the space beside him.

I put my hand on his shoulder and said, "I really liked your dad, Danny. He was a great guy."

"Yeah," he said, his voice steady, his serious eyes meeting mine. "He fought really hard."

"Yes, he did," I said, trying, but failing, to solve the equation that had a nine-year-old talking like a grown up. My eyes burned. The real possibility of crying was closing in. I needed to wrap this up.

I looked to the far side of the room again. The receiving line seemed to have broken up for the time being, and Carol stood by herself. A good opportunity for us to step in and talk to her without having to make polite conversation with all the relatives we didn't know. Leaving the kids where they were, Chris and I walked over to Carol. I hugged her before speaking. She felt too thin. Her face was pale, but her eyes were dry. More than anything, she looked exhausted. Chris hugged her too.

"We're so sorry," he began.

"Thank you," she said.

"How are you doing?" I asked. It felt absurd to voice the question, but I genuinely wanted to know.

"I'm okay," she said. "It's been a hell of a year," she added with a stilted laugh that didn't carry the ring of a laugh at all.

"I know," I said. But I didn't fully know. I only knew pieces.

I willed myself to look at the casket. Dave had been a big guy, always carrying a bit of a beer belly before he got sick. The wisp of a person resting on the satin cushion didn't look like Dave. I wondered if that made it easier or harder for Carol to be next to him. I'd never understood the concept of "viewing." I knew that some people needed that kind of visual closure, but the morbid reality of standing around a dead body, aware that nothing of the person it had once carried was still there, made me want to run for the nearest exit.

Another couple I vaguely recognized as parents from one of the kids' schools approached, and Chris and I took our cue to motion to our kids and prep for exit. As we turned to go, Carol leaned over to me suddenly and whispered next to my ear, "He died in my arms." I sensed a need in her words—a desperation for someone to know this critical detail. I hugged her again without saying anything. She wasn't looking for a response.

Will and Lily met us at the doorway leading back to the outer corridor. Their faces were unreadable. Without talking, we hurried out the same double doors we entered a few minutes earlier and retraced our steps along the cracked sidewalk to our parked car.

"Well, that's over," Lily said once she buckled into her seat. She kicked off the ballet flats, stretched her feet over the middle console to the front, and flexed her toes.

I stared out the window and glimpsed the jacketless man leaning against the railing. He exhaled a stream of smoke into the air and watched, unmoving, as Chris pulled the car into the line of traffic that headed toward Main Street.

A year later, I felt the same gripping sadness as I chatted with Carol in the soccer parking lot.

"Did you guys go away at all?" I asked and hugged my sweatshirt closer against the ever-chillier air.

"No big trips," she said. "But Dan and Melissa both went away to camp for a week." She paused and looked back toward the girls. Melissa jogged up the field, passing the ball back and forth with Gabby, another friend of Will's from school. It looked like a one-touch drill of some kind. "It was bereavement camp," Carol added almost under her breath, "but, hey, they loved it."

I didn't respond right away. My mind rewound to all the moments when I'd yearned for someone to understand and share in my experience when I was a teenager facing the uncertainty of my dad's illness. How lonely it felt to never be able to talk about it. I could imagine the relief Melissa and Danny must have felt at their camp knowing that everyone they were with knew what it was like. After a minute, I said, "I think you're making good choices for them, Carol. I bet it helped to be around other kids who've faced similar losses."

"I think so," she said. She looked in the direction of the field. "Did Will have to do that CD project last week? Missy actually asked to use pictures of Dave for it. That's the first time in a year that she's wanted to look at anything about him."

I looked over at Melissa again. She and the other girls were talking and laughing on the sidelines while they took a water break. Keep letting it out, Melissa, my thoughts urged. Holding in all that sadness will tear you apart.

"That's a good first step, right?" I said turning back to Carol.

"Yeah ..." Her voice faded on the word. She stared out the front windshield into the gathering evening dusk. She shifted her gaze back to mine and let out a hollow laugh, saying, "I can't believe this is my life. It just sucks, you know? Cancer sucks."

I nodded.

Cancer did suck. It was a cruel, cruel disease. I knew it was horrible. I knew it devastated and tore families to shreds. I knew.

And still, I'd always wished my father had been diagnosed with cancer instead of HIV.

Then, I could have said to people: "My dad has cancer."

Instead, because he was diagnosed with a disease that a majority of society judged unacceptable, I couldn't say anything at all.

Stigma

"Too BAD WE can't bottle up Ebola and set it loose in the Middle East."

These words slipped past the intensity of my concentration, and, for a few slow seconds, I didn't register their meaning. They fought for space amidst the more-focused thoughts and images I wrestled to bring to the half-filled page on my MacBook's screen. When I did register their meaning, my fingers stopped typing mid-sentence, and I looked around, not convinced I'd heard right.

My "office," the coffee shop in downtown Nashua where I liked to work, buzzed with weekend patrons fueling up on lattes and cappuccinos. I was planted in my favorite spot: a high, round table tucked in the corner by the bank of tall windows overlooking the front sidewalk. The back-and-forth traffic at the counter was far enough away that I didn't get easily distracted.

Beside me, a small group comprising three middle-aged men and one woman surrounded a rectangular wooden table. One man wore a bright yellow t-shirt that flaunted a coiled rattlesnake and the defiant *Don't Tread on Me* motto. The rest wore shirts adorned with various representations of the stars and stripes. The woman's long, graying hair partially covered a distressed image of the American flag, its edges ending in a swept brushstroke effect.

This patriotic crew was a familiar fixture on these Saturday mornings when I managed to escape the house to write. They gathered to sip coffee from oversized mugs and dissected the country's failures. Their ongoing discussions about President Obama's gun control legislation and how his "socialist agenda" threatened our personal freedoms sounded a lot like the daily commentary on the Fox News Channel. Most of the time, I tuned them out with acoustic guitar strumming through my earbuds, but I'd forgotten to remind Pandora that I was "still listening," so my station had paused long enough for this snippet of their conversation to reach me.

I wasn't sure which of the men made the Ebola comment, but Mr. Don't Tread on Me ran with it. "That would teach those Muslim Isis bastards a lesson," he said, a nauseating arrogance charging his words. "God's wrath in full force."

A sour taste filled my mouth. I steadied my hands on the table, the tile mosaic cool against my fingers. This kind of ignorant vitriol was nothing new, but linking disease and God's punishment struck in me a painful chord.

It wasn't the first time during those months in late 2014 that a haze of déjà vu had drifted into my consciousness. Like everyone else, I'd been swept up in the obsessive attention that media outlets had given to Ebola's rapid spread in West Africa. I'd glued my eyes to the television and watched the sensational images flash across the screen of health care workers, clad in yellow HAZMAT suits, treating the first cases of the outbreak in North America. I'd heard the stories of parents pulling children from a middle school in Mississippi because the principal had traveled to Zambia, even though it was a country at the center of the African continent—a thousand miles away from the primary areas of concern.

Will, who played trumpet in the Nashua High School North marching band, came home from the Friday night football game the previous week and reported, "A group of fans on the other team were chanting, 'North has Ebola! Nashua has Ebola!'" The uncertainty on his face told me he wasn't sure whether it was a big deal.

"You're kidding," I'd said, feeling a little sick. "Did anybody do anything?"

"Their cheerleaders came over and apologized after the game."

With new mandates for quarantines and heightened levels of caution surrounding a virus that was known only to spread through bodily fluids when a patient was symptomatic, I'd observed a growing panic. A panic that fed on people's fear of what wasn't known and bred suspicion and stigma. A panic I recognized.

In the 1980s and mid-1990s, few people were apologizing for their ignorant, often misguided, and cruel responses to the growing AIDS pandemic. My dad learned of his infection in December of 1985 when, eight months after his surgery, a public health official identified the blood he'd been given as contaminated, and his doctors tested him to confirm the disastrous news. We lived then in a frightened society. A society that largely believed that people diagnosed with HIV were responsible for their own infection.

In a feature piece in the fall of 1985, *Time* magazine called people with AIDS "The New Untouchables." Inconsistent and conflicting messages of how HIV spread made people afraid of even coming into contact with someone infected with the virus. When one child in a New York City school was identified as having AIDS, crowds of parents picketed the streets of New York wearing shirts reading: *No AIDS in Our Schools* and called on the city to pass legislation banning the child admission. In an op-ed for the *New York Times*, commentator William F. Buckley, Jr. called for all HIV-positive persons to be branded, saying, "Everyone detected with AIDS should be tattooed." In Canada, members of groups with names like "Citizens Demanding the Right to Know" spoke in public forums and accused medical experts of hiding the truth about the disease. Officials from the Canadian government's health department debated protective measures as radical as publicly identifying all individuals who tested positive for HIV and enforcing mandatory quarantines to protect the general population. Many people known to be HIV positive or have AIDS were fired by their employers, evicted by their landlords, and shunned by their neighbors. Because of systemic inequities in community structures and healthcare, and the exclusion of Black voices from the public conversations and education initiatives, communities of color faced disproportionate infection rates. And since that time, those disparities have only deepened.

And then there were those, much like Mr. Don't Tread on Me's posture about Ebola in the coffee shop, who claimed AIDS as a weapon of God's wrath. The evangelical Christian right was one of the loudest voices of discrimination in the 1980s. Jerry Falwell, an influential Southern Baptist preacher, televangelist, and founder of the Moral Majority, which was a political action group associated with the Republican Party whose agenda reflected fundamentalist Christian concepts of morality, declared, "AIDS is not just God's punishment for homosexuals; it is God's punishment for the society that tolerates homosexuals." Conservative commentator Pat Buchanan, a close advisor to President Reagan, called AIDS "Nature's revenge on homosexuals." This message of hatred and intolerance trickled down and established a church culture where those infected with HIV, condemned for bringing on their own demise, were not only unwelcome, they were also denied the care and compassion that Christianity ardently preached.

Elements of this harmful theology played a considerable role in shaping my family's isolated trajectory. As a devout Christian, my father struggled to reconcile his situation with society's and the evangelical church's perceptions of his disease and its causes. He'd grown up in a fundamentalist church tradition that believed homosexuality was a sinful lifestyle choice. The homophobia that sprouted from that belief was fixed in him. As a young girl, I took that belief for granted because I knew nothing else. Throughout my childhood, I learned from him and that same church tradition, the faith platitude, "Love the sinner; hate the sin," that conveniently allowed me and other Christians I knew to pass judgment (under the guise of "Christian love") on members of the LGBTQ+ community. My father's implicit and explicit messages about homosexuality—including a tendency to indelicately point out the friends in my brothers' circles who he concluded were "homos"—amplified in our household the shame and deviance that many in the 1980s mainstream culture already associated with the gay community. My heart hurts for my brother David who, for eighteen years, lived closeted in that environment, unable to find safe space to be himself amidst these barriers. My family's social network was insular, making it easy to diminish and condemn a group that felt far-removed from our lives. Even when the reality of my dad's HIV status had the potential to bridge that separation, he could not acknowledge the connection because he was entrenched in the mindset of the religious institutions that blamed the gay community for the spread of HIV. As a result of delayed and apathetic public and government response to the disease, support mechanisms for people living with HIV/AIDS were established almost exclusively by activists within the gay community. These mechanisms seemed beyond my father's reach, and any nod in the direction of their activism antithetical to his religious upbringing. His prejudice also fueled his fears that his personal reputation was at risk. What if people believed he was gay?

In the twenty-plus years since David came out to our family, I've watched my mother's beliefs about homosexuality pivot far away from the fundamentalist views she and my father espoused when I was younger, as her experience and understanding has broadened. I'd like to think Dad would be different today, too, but the chance to know was taken from us before his evolution had the opportunity to begin. I do know that when he received his diagnosis, Dad saw AIDS and all of its associations as threats to everything he valued.

Even though he was an accomplished physician, Dad felt disempowered by the limitations of his and the greater health system's knowledge about the facts of HIV. AIDS was a mystery. The only certainties were that the disease spread at a rapid rate and there was no cure. He expected that, like most patients he knew or knew about, he could die at any time, in any number of terrible ways. He was unwilling to chance infecting his patients, and he made the painful choice to end his medical practice, taking an advisory position in a national medical-legal association. He refused to allow his family to endure any form of ostracism because of his HIV status. His illness would be a secret from almost everyone. A secret we'd all keep.

We didn't know that Dad would live past that first year, or for the next ten years. And we didn't know that long after the secret was exposed, we'd continue to carry its silence.

Starting to Crack
2012

SCRAPING OFF THE residue of thirty-year-old secrets, it turns out, is not so easy.

"It takes courage to be vulnerable," Dr. B said and fixed me with his steady gaze.

Well, crap, I thought, and avoided his eyes. My thumbnail started a pattern of curved dents on my Styrofoam Dunkin' Donuts cup. My courage meter was at an all-time low, and the idea of opening up to this guy, even after almost four months of coming to his office, still made my pulse quicken and my muscles stiffen, poising my body to flee.

But there was a part of me that wanted to. A part of me that knew the old way of dealing with thorny emotions (ignoring them) wasn't working anymore. And that part kept me coming to this space, week after week, clutching the cup of tea that served as my therapy security blanket, to sit on the center cushion of this brown leather couch and inch closer and closer to painful memories from my past.

I blamed my friend Gretchen.

A few months earlier, we'd been chatting on the phone and at the end of our conversation, she mentioned that she was heading out to the spa. "Not really the spa," she qualified with a laugh. "I'm actually going to therapy."

"Okay—what?"

"Going to therapy is like going to the spa, only better because you get to talk about yourself the whole time!" she said. Her enthusiasm was contagious.

I liked the spa, I thought. Sign me up.

What I'd since discovered was this: therapy was nothing like the spa.

Unless it was one of those Asian fish spas where tiny carp nibbled the dead skin off your feet. Except instead of carp, they were razor-teethed piranha. And they didn't nibble your feet. They tore the flesh from your body in giant, agonizing chunks.

Clearly, Gretchen needed a new spa.

"Closing off your emotions is less risky," Dr. B continued shifting position in his chair, uncrossing and re-crossing his legs. "It's safer."

Damn right it's safer, I thought, tightening my hold on the cup and focusing my attention on a rogue thread that didn't belong on the cuff of Dr. B's pants. I liked safe. I liked knowing what to expect. Knowing what to expect helped light my path so I knew where to step. How to move forward. Do what needed to be done. Function.

But lately, I'd been stumbling. I couldn't seem to find my way forward because the past was dragging me back, determined to get my attention whether I wanted to give it or not. "Look at me," it kept saying. "I matter."

My resistance was trying to hold strong, but I was cracking. And despite my efforts to demonstrate otherwise, Dr. B knew it. I fretted about the gears of psychology rotating in his head and worried he'd read into my obvious discomfort and get all therapy-energized by the idea that we were on the verge of a breakthrough. That was why we kept circling back to this conversation about vulnerability and courage and risk. I hated vulnerability and courage and risk. I wrapped my arms around my body in a defensive move.

An unexpected image entered my mind. A snapshot of a five-inch decorative dish on my bedroom dresser at home. A delicate, cream-colored china plate with gold-leaf edging. In its center was a painting of a charming stone cottage, walls traced with crawling ivy. Pink and white blossoms congregated in the surrounding grounds. Beneath the painting, inscribed in curling letters, was the first verse of William Wordsworth's poem, "The Lesser Celandine."

There is a Flower, the Lesser Celandine
That shrinks, like many more, from cold and rain;
And, the first moment that the sun may shine,
Bright as the sun himself, 'tis out again!

With the thought that I could potentially steer the conversation toward a different path, I decided to launch into a story about this plate and tell Dr. B about its history.

The Christmas morning I was a senior in college, I'd unwrapped a small box with a tag that read: *To Meligans, Love Dad* written in his slanting handwriting. The plate was nestled inside, surrounded by green tissue paper. I traced the inscription with my fingers and fought back tears. I looked to where Dad sat on the couch, his arm resting across my mother's shoulders, an expectant smile playing on his lips.

"I found it in a little antique store on the South Shore this fall," he said, his chest puffing in self-satisfaction.

"You remembered," I breathed, a feeling, gentle like a summer breeze, warming me from the inside.

"I remembered," he said.

Earlier that year, when I was home for summer break, I'd sat next to Dad in a dark theater watching *A River Runs Through It*, a movie set in Missoula, Montana, around the time of World War I. It's the story of a Presbyterian minister and his two sons—Norman, played by Craig Sheffer, and Paul, played by Brad Pitt. Their relationships are complicated and ultimately tragic, but throughout the film as their lives travel divergent paths, the boys and their father maintain a fragile connection through their love of fly-fishing on the Black Foot River. My dad was a fly fisherman, and the cinematography that captured the beauty of sun-gilded fishing lines casting in a perfect rhythm over rippling streambeds was right up his alley.

In one scene, Norman, the good, reliable son who never captures his father's attention the way his rebellious brother, Paul, can, stands outside his father's study and listens to him read from a book of poetry. Norman steps in and completes a line of the poem. His father continues reading, and the two volley the words back and forth for a few more lines. Then they finish the verse together. In this moment, they've discovered a way to communicate.

The poem is William Wordsworth's "Intimations of Immortality," a poem I memorized that spring when I took an elective class on the romantic poets—Wordsworth, Coleridge, Byron, Shelley, and Keats. As the scene played out on the screen, I leaned over and whispered the words to the poem in Dad's ear in tandem with the actors. "Though nothing can bring back the hour of splendor in the grass, of glory in the flower; we will grieve not, rather find strength in what remains behind." Dad turned in his seat, a look of surprise and then pride lighting his features. "Wordsworth is my favorite," I said softly when the scene ended. Dad put his hand over mine on the armrest between us and squeezed.

"This little gift on Christmas morning spoke to something huge," I told Dr. B. "I felt like Dad understood what I cared about. What really mattered to me. It was this tangible sign of his approval, you know?"

Dr. B nodded, but I could tell by the question lodged in the curve of his brows that he was on the hunt for this tale's connection to our conversation about vulnerability and courage.

Another scene materialized in my head, and I wanted to kick myself when I realized I hadn't steered off the previous conversation's path at all.

An early spring afternoon during my final semester midterms, I was functioning on little sleep and a lot of caffeine and running especially late for my Victorian Lit exam. I rushed around my room in the dorm apartment I shared with three other girls, trying to find a book. I finally spotted it on the cluttered shelf of my college-issue desk, right next to where that Wordsworth plate sat in its wooden stand. I grabbed the book and bumped the plate. My reflexes weren't fast enough and it crashed down on the desk and shattered. Shards of porcelain scattered across the papers littering the desk's surface. I turned away, unable to register the destruction. Stabs of a pain I hardly ever acknowledged threatened, but I shut them down. I grabbed my bag and walked out the door without a word to my roommate, Sherri, who reclined on her bed with a heavy anatomy textbook resting on her knees.

In the hour and a half I was gone, Sherri took a trip to the college bookstore, bought Super Glue, and with a precision I still couldn't comprehend, pieced the plate back together. Before heading off to her exam, she left it propped back in its stand.

I was exhausted by the time I walked back through the door. The essay I'd written on the Victorian Ideal still revolved in my brain. I wanted to ignore the mess of the room, the damage on my desk, and climb into my bed and switch everything off. That was my plan when I caught sight of the plate. Cracks barely visible, it waited for me on the shelf. I stared at it, taking a moment to understand what I was seeing before a strangled sound escaped my throat. My knees buckled, and I collapsed onto the floor. I let the sobs come. Grief and gratitude intertwined, a taut rope that pulled long subdued emotions to the surface. With my face buried in my hands, I stayed there for a while.

After that, though, as ridiculous as it sounds, I was afraid to touch the plate. While it rested undisturbed on the shelf, it was safe and to any outside observer appeared whole. But I knew the truth: the plate was still broken. I knew that if I touched it, it would come apart in my hands, and I wouldn't have the wherewithal to know how to put it back together myself.

"That's what I feel like when we start talking about those early days of facing Dad's diagnosis," I admitted to Dr. B. "The frightened young girl from then is still alive somewhere inside me now. And she's so fragile. I know because any time we get close to her in our conversations, I feel her breaking. The glue I've smeared on her splintered pieces for thirty years starts pulling free, exposing the cracks." I stopped and again curled my body into a protective hug. I couldn't voice my next thought. *What happens if she shatters, and I don't know how to put her back together again?*

Dr. B sat back in his upholstered chair, his thumb and index finger tracing the shape of his bearded chin in the unnerving way of his that I'd come to understand was how he gave my words room to breathe. "What are you afraid of?" he asked finally.

In response to his question, my heart beat faster, and my breath felt trapped in my chest. Flashes of memory spun through my mind, a kaleidoscope of shifting moments when the well of sadness felt bottomless and the shadows of uncertainty and dread hovered too close. Those same feelings felt too close now.

The sky was dark out the window over Dr. B's shoulder. Menacing clouds roiled across its expanse. A storm moved in. Raindrops pelted the window and echoed in the quiet office.

He asked again: "What are you afraid of, Melanie?"

I sighed the air from my lungs and didn't brush away the tears that stung my eyes. I stopped fighting the remembered moments when I had no way of voicing the terror I felt.

"Everything," I said.

Uncertainty and Dread
1985

THE WEEK BEFORE Christmas, Dad took a day-trip to Nova Scotia. "Dad's doctor needs him to have some important tests," Mom said. I thought that maybe it had something to do with Dad's heart because he went to the same hospital in Halifax where he'd had his surgery. But when he got back later that night, they didn't tell me the results. They did, I know now, tell Michael and Mark, but they didn't say anything to me.

Instead, they kept packing our things into cardboard boxes, getting ready for our cross-country move in two weeks to Ontario. Dad was starting a new job as a medical advisor for the Canadian Medical Protective Association—a temporary career shift he'd chosen when his cardiologist warned the stress of his surgical practice was too much for his heart.

They acted like everything was normal as they prepped for Christmas. Yet, even though they wrapped presents and made cookies and shopped for the Christmas dinner fixings, even though Mom prepared Christmas punch and appetizers on Christmas Eve, even though Dad played my favorite carols on the upright piano— "Silent Night" and "O, Come All Ye Faithful" and "Joy to the World"— even though they said "Merry Christmas" on Christmas morning and passed out presents wrapped in shiny paper from under the twinkling tree, and even though they laughed and pasted wide smiles on their faces and did everything we always did to make the season bright, an ominous cloud hung over everything.

When they didn't think I was looking, they met each other's gazes, their lips in tight lines, brows creasing in the middle. Tears pooled in Mom's eyes again and again, followed by her excuses that she was "just feeling a little sad because this was our last Christmas in Moncton." The false brightness of her tone made me feel like she was lying. My parents' hushed conversations stopped abruptly when I walked into the room, but not before I heard the distress in their voices.

Trauma researchers say that our brains can hide experiences to protect us from having to relive them. To protect us from overwhelming fear or stress that is tied to them. Sometimes those experiences remain hidden forever. Maybe this is what happened to me because even though *how* I knew remains a baffling hole in my memory, I knew.

Dad had AIDS.

Four days after Christmas, on the eve of our move, in the dark of my bedroom, feeling the press of a threat I could name but could not understand, all I wanted to do was un-know.

My back pushed into the wooden headboard, and I squeezed my knees against my chest. I clutched my bedspread to my chin. I stared into the night, my eyes burning with the strain of trying to glimpse the thing hiding in the dark, hovering over the new emptiness of my bare shelves and vacant drawers. All my belongings were packed away and sealed with wide strips of tape in the boxes stacked and waiting for the moving van's arrival the next day.

The air escaped my lips in shallow gasps. I tried to shut down the blur of frightening thoughts and images that cartwheeled through my brain as I took inventory of what I knew about AIDS. On the news, I'd seen the stories of people, mostly gay men, developing horrible illnesses because of the virus. I'd seen the magazine covers in news-stands describing this disease with words like *Plague* and *Epidemic* and *Threat*. I'd heard of picketers lining the streets outside of schools and carrying signs with hateful slogans to keep away children who'd tested positive for the disease. I'd listened, unsure how to react, to some boys in my eighth-grade class taunt other kids on the playground with the words: "Careful not to get too close to *him*, you might get AIDS!"

The one thing I didn't want to know, I knew for certain: There was no cure.

When I was four or five, I was convinced a bad man with a machete lived under my bed. Certain that if I stepped straight down next to the mattress, he'd cut my bare feet off at the ankles, I made a plan. I'd jump out at an angle, at least two feet past the edge, and as soon as my feet hit the plush pink carpet, I'd dash to the door. I did it for years. I have no idea how I thought up such a grisly image, but its origin could probably be traced back to my two older brothers. The thing was, I didn't worry about anything else this machete-wielding man might do. As I lay tucked into my gingham sheets, the thought never crossed my mind that he could have any other evil plans percolating. I wasn't afraid. I knew he had only one goal: my feet. And I'd figured out how to outsmart him and protect myself.

But AIDS was a different danger. Mysterious. Complicated. Unpredictable. There was no way for me to make a protective plan against what was coming. No way for me to stop the fear.

I glanced at the dim outline of my closed door. I could open that door, I thought. I could step out into the hallway, tiptoe the fifteen feet to my parents' bedroom, knock, and ask them for help. Ask them for help to fend off the terror I was feeling. But I wasn't supposed to know about Dad. They'd left me out. Had they told my older brothers? Nobody was talking. An unsure guilt from carrying a secret that was not mine rose up and made me hesitate. Kept me pinned to the mattress.

I tried, instead, to pray.

"Tell me what to do," I pleaded into the inky darkness.

Even though I couldn't see past the night, I pictured the walls of my bedroom. Rainbows. Pastel arcs reaching out from puffy white clouds scattered across a pale blue sky above a strip of white molding that traced the perimeter of the space. "You can decorate your new bedroom however you want," Mom and Dad had promised three years ago when I was ten and we'd moved to this large house on Ammon Road. The new house was still inside the Moncton city limits, but far enough away from our old neighborhood, Centennial Place, and I had to switch schools right before grade six. My parents' diplomatic gesture to ease the transition worked well.

"That one," I'd said when I'd seen the sample strip of this pattern hanging next to the rolls of wallpaper at the paint store.

I loved rainbows. I always had.

I remembered sitting on a square of blue carpet on a linoleum floor in a preschool Sunday school classroom. I was in a circle of children, my legs crossed, my shiny, patent leather shoes tucked beneath my thighs. I smoothed the hem of my flowered dress over my knees. I remembered my Sunday school teacher's wide smile and her long, brown hair that fell in waves at her shoulders. I loved her high-heeled shoes that matched her dresses. She placed colorful cutouts on the wide, flannel board propped up on an easel while she told my class a story about a man named Noah and a giant flood. So many years later, I could still see the wooden ark with its curved hull and the long, wide ramp leading into its depths. I remembered the unlikely pairs of animals trailing up that ramp – giraffes, elephants, lions, hippos, zebras, bears, kangaroos, mice, ostriches, alligators, turtles. I remembered the cutout of Noah, his white beard almost reaching his feet, and the cutouts of his wife and his children. I remembered a snowy dove carrying a branch in its beak flying through cotton ball clouds and splayed rays of sunlight. "A Bible sky," Dad always called it.

And I heard my Sunday school teacher's animated words: "And when God brought Noah and his family safely through the flood waters and the ark settled on dry land, they opened the doors and the animals all ran out to fill the world again. Noah prayed to God to thank him for keeping them safe, and God spoke to Noah and said, 'Look up into the sky.'"

Miss Shelly paused for effect, her smile even wider, and then set the last image on the board—a bright rainbow that arched over the entire scene. She finished the story. "God had a plan for Noah. God sent this rainbow to him and his family as a special promise called a covenant. He promised Noah that there would never be another flood to destroy the earth. The rainbow would always be a reminder of this promise."

She asked us to raise our hands if we'd ever seen a rainbow. Everyone's hand shot up.

"I saw one when we went camping before," one boy said, his arm still waving.

"There was one in the sky right after it thundered and lightninged," the girl beside me said and her voice bubbled with excitement. "My dad took a bunch of pictures because it was sunny on one side of the sky and dark and cloudy on the other."

Miss Shelly knelt so her face was level with ours, an invitation to lean in, to absorb this lesson. "Well, the next time you see a rainbow, I want you to remember that God loves you." She tapped each of our folded knees, repeating the words, "and you and you and you" with each soft touch. "Remember that whenever there's a storm, there will always be a bright new day on the other side. God has a plan for you. That's God's promise. God never breaks a promise."

I listened to Miss Shelly's hushed voice, and I believed her. I looked at the rainbow on the flannel board, and I tucked this story into my mind and my heart and let it become a barometer for how I reacted when things didn't go my way. God never broke a promise. God had a plan. There would always be a brighter day.

That's what I'd believed then. That's what I wanted to believe in the moment I lay alone in the dark. We'd weathered the storm when Dad had his heart attack, I thought. We'd done the hard thing already, and Dad got better.

After his quadruple bypass eight months earlier, I'd watched his strength return as he plodded the slow path to recovery. The distance of his doctor-mandated "hikes" lengthened day by day: To the end of the front walk. To the top of the driveway. To the neighbor's house and back. He made steady progress and eventually walked long miles in one direction on our country road with Sandy, our Shetland sheepdog, trotting at his side.

With relief, I watched his slumped shoulders start to straighten again. Watched the long, angry scars on his chest and leg begin to fade, covered over by his dark hair. Watched him make optimistic preparations for this upcoming change in career, knowing with everyone else that, despite his cardiologist's warnings about the stresses of his surgical practice, sooner than later he'd return to the operating room, to the work he loved. "Thank you," I prayed to my God of unbroken promises. "Thank you for bringing him back."

I even accepted our impending move away from my friends, from everything I knew, as a necessary step toward our bright new day.

But an invisible danger had entered my world and pierced the light. AIDS. How did AIDS fit into the story?

I pressed my knuckles to my lips to stop their trembling, desperate to believe that God was still listening to my prayers.

"AIDS is God's punishment." I'd heard these words rippling through my evangelical Christian community. Until that moment, though, I hadn't paid attention to their meaning. There was no reason to think they had anything to do with me or with my father.

"What do I do?" I whispered, an added fierceness underwriting my words, trying to push back my swelling doubts. None of it made sense. Why would God punish Dad? Punish me?

"Give me an answer," I prayed. "Tell me the plan."

"Please." This final word waited, suspended in the air.

I waited with it, straining my eyes to see into the night.

Silence.

The Language of Tragedy

RAUCOUS CHATTER FILLED my social studies classroom as my classmates and I bustled in from our lunch break and made our way to our desks. I reached into the small paper bag of penny candy from my trip to Mac's convenience store and popped the last of my Swedish Berries into my mouth. Taking my seat, I savored the chewy sweetness. A novelty of my new school setting was the opportunity to leave the grounds at lunchtime since most of the students lived within walking distance. The bus kids and others, like me, who lived beyond the school's immediate neighborhoods, ate in our homerooms, but we were free to venture outside if there was time before the afternoon bell.

Today, as I'd stuffed the half-eaten remnants of my lunch back into my locker in the hallway outside of our class, Nicole, a petite, bubbly girl I'd started to get to know, had walked over, put her hand on my arm and said, "A few of us are going to run down to Mac's for a treat. Want to come?"

"Sure," I said, trying not to sound too eager, but feeling a swell of excitement pulse beneath my skin as I shrugged my ski jacket over my chunky, oversized sweater and followed her out the front entrance. I walked with her and two other girls from my homeroom—Stephanie and Crystal—up the snow-scattered sidewalk that flanked Greenbank Road, trying to keep my flimsy Keds from getting wet in the slushy puddles.

Though all of the kids in grade eight at Greenbank Middle School had been friendly since I'd arrived three weeks earlier following Christmas vacation, I still felt very much the "new girl." I struggled to find my place in the well-established social circles. Most of my classmates had been together since kindergarten. It didn't help that I wasn't living in the part of the city that fed this school district. While waiting for our house in Moncton to sell, my parents had rented a small, furnished bungalow in an older neighborhood, a ten-minute drive away. They'd enrolled Mark, David, and me in schools in Nepean—a suburb of Ottawa where they planned to buy a home once ours sold. Michael was back in Moncton, living with family friends, finishing out his last six months of high school. Everything familiar had been upended, replaced by a new reality, one that felt alien and shaky. Talking and laughing with Nicole and the other girls during our quick trip to the store had presented me with a rare flash of steadiness.

Just after I sat down, our social studies teacher, Mr. Collins, entered the room and walked to the front of the class. Behind him, the green chalkboard was covered in vocabulary and dates about the colonies of British North America written in his messy script. Maps of Canada and the US with large pointing arrows covered the corkboards. Mr. Collins leaned his lanky frame against his desk and raked his fingers through his dark, curly hair, before clearing his throat. Probably in his late thirties, Mr. Collins was an energetic guy whose dry sense of humor and contagious enthusiasm for learning made his class my favorite in the weeks I'd been there. That day as he stood before us, though, the uncharacteristic slouch of his shoulders and the dullness around his eyes gave us pause, and an uncertain quiet descended over my classmates and me. He cleared his throat again.

"Something's happened," he began, his voice thick with the weight of whatever he was about to say.

Dread lurched into my stomach. I clamped down hard on my back teeth, gripped my hands together in my lap, and waited.

"About thirty minutes ago, when the space shuttle launched from Cape Canaveral in Florida, something happened." He struggled to extend his words to the specifics. "There was some kind of malfunction ... an explosion." His voice cracked.

"What kind of explosion?" a boy, whose name I couldn't remember, asked, his question tinged with alarm.

"A catastrophic one," Mr. Collins said gently, and his eyes reddened. "The news reports are saying that everyone on board is presumed dead."

A few gasps erupted around the room, and I scanned the faces of my classmates, each one shadowed with a mixture of shock and sadness. Just the day before, Mr. Collins was telling us about how excited he was to see a teacher—"Not just any teacher, but a *social studies* teacher," he proudly emphasized—travel to space for the first time. It was Christa McAuliffe, the New Hampshire high school teacher chosen to be the first participant in the NASA Teacher in Space Program and the first private citizen to join an expedition, and her presence on the seven-person crew of the *Challenger*, that made this launch unique and captured our collective interest in Canada too.

"It's such a terrible tragedy," Mr. Collins said. "I'll be honest. I'm feeling pretty bad about it all. I'm sure you guys must be feeling some of that too. If you want to talk about it, we definitely can." He sat on the top of his metal desk and picked up his miniature globe, spinning it absently.

"Did you actually see it blow up?" asked the same boy who'd spoken earlier. This kid's need to gather the intricate facts to piece the story together reminded me of the way my little brother David processed things.

"I wasn't watching the launch live," Mr. Collins said. "But we turned on the news in the teachers' room at lunch when Principal Eaton came in and told us what happened, and we saw the replay a few minutes later."

"Do you think the astronauts' families watched it happen?" Nicole asked from her seat next to me, alarm shaking her voice. Until her question, my mind hadn't traveled beyond the seven people on board of the shuttle and what they'd experienced, but now all I could think about was how terrible it must have felt for the spectators on the ground to witness the disaster. TV news footage I'd see replayed again and again over the next few days would make those thoughts real as the camera's lens captured not just the explosion and the forked plumes of smoke and fire against the blue sky, but close up images of people in the crowd as the horrific recognition of what they were seeing registered on their faces.

"I know they were," Mr. Collins answered, "And I know that a lot of students in the US were watching the launch live from their classrooms. Mrs. McAuliffe's students were. Her whole school was." He stopped and looked away before swiping his hand across his eyes. "That kind of grief is hard to think about. It's such a huge loss ..." his words petered out into another uncertain quiet.

The air in the room had shifted, a new heaviness saturating the space. I felt it in my body, in my limbs, adding to a weight that was already there, pressing hard against unnamed feelings I'd been carrying around for weeks. But now, these words Mr. Collins was using—"tragedy," "grief," "loss"—gave me, for the first time, a language I could attach to them.

My family had suffered an explosion too. Our charted path had been obliterated by the news of my father's HIV infection, and I felt lost in the aftermath, trying, but failing, to recognize who we now were.

We'd become invisible in this new city, no longer known by the reputation of our name and my father's good work. In so many bewildering ways, our life had shrunk. Our rental was a fraction of the size of the sprawling, split-level house we'd left behind in Moncton. Cramped with outdated furniture that wasn't ours and surrounded by unfriendly neighbors, nothing about it felt like home. Mark didn't even have a real bedroom, but had settled, instead, for some space of his own in the windowless basement. I missed my rainbow room and my big yard bordered by the dense woods where I'd loved to wander, casting myself part of whimsical scenes from my favorite books, content to live for hours in my imagination. These days, my mind was a frightening place, too often occupied by awful images of what might be ahead for us, for Dad.

I ached for the comfort of my friends and our daily rituals of calling one another as soon as we arrived home after school to plan meet-ups at different houses. Here, there was no one to call, and I walked through the days, timid and awkward, desperate to decode the subtext that would help me fit in with this group of strangers.

Michael's departure from our family circle had come too soon, and without his gregarious presence, we were incomplete. I imagined how lonely it must be for him to be cut off from our present experience, kept separate by so many miles and the too-painful things left unsaid in phone conversations and letters.

I longed to see Dad's face light up the way it used to when he'd swoop in for dinner in between surgeries, eager to hear about our days, and energized by the challenge and excitement of his own. In his new job, he spent dreary hours entombed in a quiet room, sitting at a desk, reading files, and trying to understand his new administrative work. At the end of each day, he seemed faded somehow.

Mom was doing everything she could to keep us busy, to help us settle in, to create some semblance of normal in circumstances that were anything but. She was hyper-focused on finding music teachers for my brothers and me, enrolling us in swimming lessons, and planning weekend outings to explore different parts of our new city. In contrast to Dad, she was in constant motion. An anxious undercurrent moved beneath her actions, and there were unsettling moments when the reassuring picture she was trying to paint over our situation showed its cracks. This week, she'd handed the car keys to Mark, who wasn't yet sixteen and didn't have a driver's license, and allowed him to chauffeur David and me the ten minutes—on the four-lane highway—to our schools before driving himself to the high school.

And yet, I said nothing, swallowing hard against my unasked questions, doing what I was expected to do, because nobody was pausing to talk to me about any of it. I didn't know whether or not my parents suspected that I'd figured some things out about Dad's health. What I did know was that they needed me to be okay. And so, for most of the time, I was.

But as I sat in that classroom and listened to Mr. Collins talk about the *Challenger* disaster, the sadness and confusion around me bumped against the churning feelings inside, and okay felt distant.

"It makes me want to cry," Stephanie said.

I expected somebody to laugh—maybe one of the boys—but nobody did. Instead, her words were met with murmurs of agreement.

"Of course, it does," Mr. Collins said. He picked up the box of tissues from his desk and rose to his feet. Walking over to Stephanie, he extended it toward her. She took one and gave him a small, grateful smile. "It's a terrible, terrible tragedy," he said again. "It makes me want to cry too." This time, he didn't brush away his tears.

Watching him, my own eyes filled. I was surprised to see a grown-up talk openly about his feelings. This, too, was unfamiliar territory. Yet, unlike the other episodes of the last few weeks, I didn't wish this one away.

And Mr. Collins wasn't expecting us to carry on with our regularly scheduled social studies lesson either. Something important had happened, and he knew we needed him to allow room for us to talk about it. The worksheets mapping the colonies we'd completed the night before would sit uncorrected for the remainder of the class period as more of my classmates asked tentative questions and let themselves feel the emotional effects of the shuttle's explosion.

As late January's white light sliced through the window, casting shards across my desk, I didn't speak. I couldn't separate all of my messy feelings into something concrete about the day's events. But I listened closely and leaned into the collective sadness, depositing some of my own there, too, if only for a while. I relaxed my hands and loosened my jaw. A soft sigh brushed past my lips.

So Little Information,
So Much Fear

I PAUSED ON the landing, my hand resting on the heavy door handle and turned to wave to Mr. Renner, my next-door neighbor. He stood on his front step, the inside light framing his silhouette, and watched to make sure I got in the house all right. "Good night," he said and turned into his entryway. Once I'd passed over the threshold and pulled the door closed, the deadbolt secured, I sifted through the bills he'd handed me on my way out. Thirty dollars. Not bad for a late night of babysitting. Especially since William and Ryan, two and four, had fallen asleep by eight. The rest of the evening, I'd luxuriated on their family room couch and watched *St. Elmo's Fire* on cable, munching the salt and vinegar chips and drinking the Coke he and Mrs. Renner had left for me.

Except for the stove light casting a glow from the kitchen, the house was dark and still. Mom and Dad didn't typically wait up when I was babysitting next door. I slipped off my Keds and padded barefoot across the tile in the front hall to turn off the light. I headed upstairs, my feet quiet on the carpet. My room was the one at the top of the stairs. I tiptoed inside, switched on my bedside lamp, and closed the door gently behind me.

The alarm clock on my desk read a little after midnight, but I was still wired from the caffeine. I grabbed a pair of worn sweats from a crumpled heap of clothes in the corner and pulled them on, along with an oversized t-shirt. Propping my pillows against the white headboard, I nestled under my down comforter. I reached for my book and found the dog-eared page in *Jane Eyre* where I'd left off and returned to the budding romance between the impressionable governess and Mr. Rochester. By twelve forty-five, my eyes were heavy and the words started to smear on the page. The details of Jane's complicated history with Mrs. Reed and the revelations of her inheritance from her uncle began to get muddy, and I decided to put down the book.

I hadn't brushed my teeth, so I climbed out of bed and opened my door, careful not to bang it against the doorstop. I slipped into the hallway and started toward the bathroom I shared with my brother David. My eyes took a few seconds to adjust to the dark, and I ran my hand along the wall to guide my path.

A soft moan stopped me midstride.

At first, I didn't realize its source, and for a few seconds, I was not certain I'd heard anything. Then, another moan sounded, louder this time, followed by a creaking mattress spring and rhythmic, heavy breathing. The sounds were coming from behind my parents' closed bedroom door.

Recognition burned through me. I was standing smack in the middle of every teenager's worst nightmare.

Indecision froze me to the spot as the now mortifyingly clear noises resonated through the hallway. If I continued to the bathroom to brush my teeth, I would alert my parents that I was awake, and chances were that one of them would come out to check on me. Totally out of the question, I decided. Heat scalded my cheeks at the thought of facing either of them in this awkward moment.

I clapped my hands over my ears, wishing I could somehow utter the la-la-las that would block the sounds now searing themselves into my brain without drawing attention to myself. I crept back to my bedroom, and in the slowest and most careful of movements, I inched the door closed. I turned off the lamp and hid beneath my comforter. I squeezed my eyes shut against the darkness, discouraging images that were trying to take shape in my mind. Embarrassment prickled my skin, but something else had opened up inside of me. A relentless and looming question that wouldn't stop repeating in my mind: What if he infects her?

I absorbed this new terror as it washed over me. The fact that I knew Dad was HIV positive had materialized for my parents without fanfare. There wasn't a moment when they formally acknowledged it, but an unspoken understanding had formed between us. On rare occasions, they'd include me in their conversations. From the few fragments I'd gathered and their answers the few times I'd been bold enough to ask about Dad's condition, I knew that after Dad found out he was HIV positive, Mom got tested too. Though the infected blood had circulated through his system for eight months before he knew about it, by some miracle, Dad hadn't passed the virus to my mother.

I knew how AIDS spread. The American Red Cross had been running a series of PSAs called "Rumors are spreading faster than AIDS" to fight against the ongoing AIDS myths. Every time I turned on the television to one of the main networks, I heard celebrities like Robert De Niro and Meryl Streep saying things like: "There isn't a single case of AIDS on record caused by casual contact." And "Find out the facts."

I knew the facts: You couldn't get AIDS from someone by shaking hands or sharing a water glass. You could get AIDS from someone by having sex and sharing needles. I knew about condoms. We'd learned about them in school during a part in health class that talked about protecting against sexually transmitted diseases, including AIDS. Just last month, on one of my favorite shows, *The Hogan Family*, Jason Bateman's character David bought a box of condoms because he was thinking of having sex with his girlfriend. And once, when I was snooping in Mom's bedside table, I found a stack of the small square packages at the back of her drawer. Then, I couldn't get beyond the mortification of the discovery to think about their use. But now, I couldn't stop thinking about them. "Remember," my health teacher cautioned, "condoms are not one hundred percent effective. The safest way to protect yourself against AIDS is to choose not to have sex."

I'd read some of the tragic public stories in the news magazines my parents subscribed to of people transmitting the disease to their partners before finding out they themselves were infected. But my parents knew about Dad's infection. Could I trust that they were doing everything they could to prevent that same kind of tragedy? I wasn't so sure. *Don't let Mom get sick. I can't lose you both. Don't risk it. Please, please, please be safe!*

I turned my face into my pillow, clapped my hands over my ears again, and, this time, I cried out, certain that no one would hear me.

The Risk Was Real

"So, WHEN DID he start displaying symptoms?"

"Sometime on Friday night, I think," Mom said, her voice calm.

"And that would have been March eighth?" The gray-suited man asked. His words were brisk. He pursed his lips in a grim line and paused to flip through the pages on the clipboard balanced on his lap. Mom had twice offered him a cup of coffee and a glass of water. He'd refused both times.

"I believe so," Mom said, answering his question about the date.

Grim Face sat in one of the wing-backed chairs in our living room. Mom sat across from him on the floral couch, her shoulders squared, her gaze steady, a polite smile plastered to her face.

"We weren't too concerned until Saturday, though," Dad said from his spot on the couch beside Mom. He had his arm propped casually behind Mom's shoulders and his other hand rested on his lap. "He began showing signs of severe dehydration: fatigue, dizziness, sunken eyes. And the vomit and diarrhea only grew more violent when we tried to get liquids into him."

"So that's when you took him to the ER?" Grim Face consulted his clipboard again and made a note in the margin next to the timeline he was creating.

"Yes. I knew he'd need IV hydration with added saline and electrolytes." Dad fell comfortably into medical speak.

It was a Saturday, almost a year after hearing I-N-T-E-R-C-O-U-R-S-E and we were in the middle of what felt like one of those police interrogations I'd seen on TV crime shows. Thirty minutes earlier, the doorbell had rung. I was reading on the couch. David was at a friend's house, and Mom and Dad were upstairs, so I'd answered the door. A thin man with a receding hairline stood on our doorstep, clipboard in one hand, ID badge in the other. "I'm an agent from the Ontario Board of Public Health. I'd like to speak to ..." he paused and glanced at his clipboard, "Orville and Dorothy Messenger."

Alarm made my body lock up, and I hesitated before inviting him in. I called upstairs to my parents.

In the three years since our move to Ottawa, my dad had never visited an Ontario physician. Every six months, he flew to Halifax to meet with his cardiologist and have his blood drawn. He explained these periodic trips away with comments about a long-standing friendship with his doctor and opportunities to reconnect with old colleagues in the Maritimes. The real reason, though, I learned later, was to make sure no health records in Ontario revealed his HIV status. Ontario had one of the strictest public health policies in Canada, and, since the country's first cases of AIDS, the Ontario government had had an ongoing debate about whether public identification of those infected with HIV should be mandatory.

"Is Mark Messenger home?" Grim Face asked when my parents entered the front hallway, the confusion at the arrival of this unexpected weekend visitor clear on their faces. "We have a report that he was treated for campylobacter at the Civic Hospital."

I exhaled. My legs steadied beneath me. This visit wasn't about Dad.

Two weeks earlier, Mark had come home for a long weekend from the University of Western Ontario where he was a pre-med student. Within hours of his arrival, he'd started feeling sick. Fever. Chills. Upset stomach. The next morning, his symptoms were worse. His abdominal pain grew severe, and his fever spiked. Mark had eaten chicken the night before coming home, and Mom and Dad suspected food poisoning. They took him to the Emergency Room, and the doctors there hydrated him with IV fluids and immediately started him on a powerful dose of antibiotics. After a few days, he recovered and returned to school.

Now, this dour agent sat in our living room dotting his i's and crossing his t's to ensure the safety of the rest of Ontario's citizens. He darted a series of questions from his checklist:

"What did Mark eat?"

"Did he share his food with anyone else?"

"Who was he in contact with?"

"Has anyone else displayed symptoms?"

"Have all the areas in the home where he made contact been sterilized?"

"Where is he now?"

"How is he feeling?"

"What kind of follow-up care has he received?"

I did not miss the irony of these questions.

I listened to my parents answer each one, impressed by their patience and composure. From where I sat on the loveseat adjacent to the couch, my eyes wandered to the gold-framed oil painting on the wall. Powerful ocean waves crashed and churned on the canvas. White-capped. Tumultuous. The force of our secret thrashed inside me. Until then, I'd never fully considered what the danger of others knowing about Dad's illness might look like, but now the risk was all-too-real and sitting across from me. How would Grim Face react if he discovered the true infectious disease inhabiting our house?

He stood up and buttoned his jacket. "That should cover things," he said. "I'll be in touch if I have any more questions." What more could he ask? I wondered. My parents ushered him to the front door.

Before he left, he turned and shook Mom's hand. Then, Dad's.

Dad closed the door and slumped against it, his body visibly shaking. His breaths came in short gasps. Mom pressed her fist to her mouth, her eyes wild. I was glued to the spot, my body rigid. I stared at them both.

For a minute, no one said anything. We listened to the car engine start up and the squeak of brakes as the agent pulled out of our driveway. Then, Dad pulled in a dramatic mouthful of air.

"Ho-ly shit," he said on the exhale, stretching the syllables like an elastic.

We burst into peals of laughter. The sound rang through the house.

The Ryan White Story, and Mine

"How were the Taylor kids last night?" Mom asked.

"Okay," I said. "A little rambunctious. Hard to settle them down for bed." I yawned. Even though I'd slept in a bit this morning instead of getting up to catch the bus, I felt wiped after arriving home past eleven the night before. I usually didn't babysit on weeknights—it was my junior year of high school, and I rarely stayed up that late—but my parents made an exception for our family friends. And since it was Monday, my homework hadn't piled yet.

I stared out the passenger window at the high bank of snow lining the road. The morning light glistened on its ice-crusted surface. Discarded Christmas trees sat atop the mounds at the ends of many of the neighborhood driveways. The crenellated grooves left behind by the plow crunched beneath the car tires as Mom turned onto Hazeldean Road toward my high school. I watched our breath exhale in puffs of fog as the heater worked to warm the air. I held my hands over the vents to keep my fingers from freezing. I was done with winter now that the holidays were over, now that 1989 was fully rung in, and, though it was only the middle of January, I was ready for spring. I yawned again.

It wasn't the umpteen games of *Go Fish!* and *Hungry Hippos* that wore me out. It wasn't filling the outlines of puppies and fairy princesses with bright Crayola colors in thick coloring books and adorning them with glittery stickers or reading multiple bedtime stories from large picture books. It was what came after I'd tucked the kids into bed.

I'd flopped down on the couch in front of the TV. Wrapped in a plaid blanket, I flipped between *MacGyver* and *Kate & Allie* before settling in to watch the ABC Movie of the Week.

As John Mellencamp's voice belted "Small Town," the screen filled with snapshots of an Indiana landscape: churches, factories, parks, schools. The Ryan White Story. How did I know that name? I couldn't remember.

It came to me fifteen minutes into the movie, when the mom from *Who's the Boss?*, now playing Ryan's mother, sat in a hospital conference room and listened to her son's doctor telling her that the recurring infection in Ryan's lungs was likely caused by a blood virus. He was the kid on the news, posing in pictures with Michael Jackson and Elton John, whose face I'd seen on the cover of *People* magazine last year. The kid with AIDS.

I wondered if my mother knew about him. Had she followed his story? Ryan White caught the nation's attention in 1986, only a few months after Dad learned of his HIV infection. Ryan, a person with hemophilia, contracted HIV from contaminated blood too. Did she know how people treated him when they found out he was infected? His small-town community of neighbors and friends, terrified by a disease no one understood, had turned against this thirteen-year-old boy and tried to keep him out of school. Far away from their children.

They'd attacked his family. In one scene, Ryan's younger sister was bullied on a bus. "My brother says your brother is a faggot!" a girl yelled. In another, set at the factory where Ryan's mother worked, a fight erupted between two workers after his mother poured coffee from a communal pot. When she assured one of the men that she didn't have AIDS and that he couldn't catch it from her, he spat back, "Yeah? How do you know?"

As I watched, a ticker tape of questions spiraled through my head. Was it the fear of these sorts of reactions that compelled my parents to keep Dad's infection a secret? Could that happen to us? Here?

Alone in my neighbors' house, I wanted to punch the OFF button on the remote, get up off the couch, and disconnect from this movie. I wanted to pretend what was happening to Ryan White—the community outrage, the isolation, the disease—had nothing to do with my family.

Pretending was easy. Dad didn't look sick. He was strong and energetic, a doctor who got up each morning, put on a suit, and went to work as a medical advisor in an office building in downtown Ottawa. He mowed the lawn and weeded the garden on weekends. He skied and ice-skated and swam and boated. He took Bailey, our golden retriever, on long walks every day. There was nothing in his manner that suggested he was different from anyone else. As far as I knew, apart from some days when he was especially tired, he was healthy.

In the movie, the actor who portrayed Ryan White, the same wide-eyed, big-eared kid who'd played that Amish boy in the movie *Witness* with Harrison Ford, was pale and thin and sickly. He struggled to breathe and spent days in the hospital with active infection.

That wasn't Dad.

But as I watched the truth of AIDS play out in vivid, cinematic detail on the screen, a new awareness funneled into my consciousness: not *yet*. I sat motionless, the blanket pulled tight against my body. I couldn't stop watching. My fists clenched against my lips, blocking the air. How would the story end?

A made-for-TV movie had a happy ending. Ryan's family moved to a new community where they found acceptance and tolerance. The final scene showed Ryan arriving at his new high school. With newspaper photographers' cameras flashing, the principal shook his hand, saying, "We're happy to have you." He led Ryan to a crowd of students who walked him toward the school building. Hope broke across his mother's face as she watched. Waving and smiling, she drove away to the catchy beat of Elton John's "I'm Still Standing."

I turned off the TV then and stared into the empty screen. A fresh dread squeezed my insides. I knew Ryan's story was not over.

The dying part just hadn't happened yet.

At home, I climbed into bed, curled into a ball, my knees once again hugged to my chest, and burrowed beneath my duvet. I couldn't stop thinking about what I'd watched. All these things didn't feel like they were supposed to belong in my world: the terrible accusations and assumptions about how Ryan had contracted HIV; hatred from both strangers and people who'd known him his whole life; people who treated him like the disease was his fault. His family lost their privacy and with it, security—something they'd always taken for granted. But the worst were the moments when Ryan was so sick he couldn't lift his head from the edge of the toilet seat. Hidden under my covers, the boding presence I'd felt with me ever since we moved from Moncton seemed so much bigger. A pressing question hammered against my skull: What's next? What's next? What's next?

This question hung on my tongue the next morning in the car on our way to school. I glanced at Mom. Her short brown permed hair was still a bit damp from her shower, and the mousse-crusted curls needed to be brushed out. Her face was smooth, even without makeup.

She steered the car down Abbeyhill Drive, approaching the entrance to the school. I drew in a shaky breath, held it, and then blurted, "Is Dad going to die?" It came out as a question, but I was not asking. The answer had been there all along. I just needed to hear it.

The car slowed. Surprise registered on Mom's face. She opened her mouth to speak and then closed it. Her lips pressed together. My question was a cavern between us.

"Mel," she began, and I could already sense in her tone that she was about to downplay, deflect, or reassure, the same way she downplayed, deflected, or reassured anytime I got brave enough to ask questions about Dad's illness.

"Just tell me." My voice was steady, but the plea behind the words made it sharp.

We approached the school. Cars crowded the rectangular parking lot out front, and students stood in clusters on the snow-packed sidewalk by the main entrance, backpacks tossed over their shoulders, their coats pulled close against the cold. Near the glass doors leading into the school, I saw my friends: Penny, John, Russell, Sunita. They were waiting for me before heading inside.

"Tell me," I said again, this time less steady, as Mom pulled up against the curb and turned in her seat toward me. "Is Dad going to die?" I turned too and faced her directly. My eyes locked on hers.

She gripped the steering wheel with her gloved hands and inhaled a measured breath. Then, speaking in a defeated voice I'd never heard before, she said, "Yes."

The single word ripped through the protective blanket that she'd wrapped around me for the last four years. It tracked into my mind, sinking like a stone to the ocean floor, where it settled for good.

"Okay." I stretched for my backpack on the floor and clutched the door handle. "Okay," I said again. I pushed the door open and climbed out into the frigid air, welcoming it into my lungs. I walked toward my friends, plastered a smile on my face, and shoved everything else back down.

Just before I entered the school, I looked back toward the car and lifted my hand to wave. Mom still gripped the wheel, her gaze trained on me. She waved back and tried to smile, but tears traced lines down her cheeks. She put the car into gear and drove away.

Putting on a Good Face

THE EVENING WAS drawing to a close. We'd arranged our folding chairs in a circle. Chuck, our youth pastor, strummed a familiar praise chorus on his guitar as the fifteen or so teenagers and handful of adults in the group took our seats. The soft, acoustic chords filled the large room and transformed the mood, urging us to shift our focus from the earlier rambunctious games and lively small-group discussions and settle into a headspace of quiet reflection. Our voices mingled with the notes, "Seek ye first the kingdom of God / And His righteousness; / And all these things shall be added unto you. / Hallelu, Hallelujah!"

To my left, my best friend Sherri harmonized, adding rich counter notes to the melody. Her dark, curly hair swung across her face as she bowed her head, lost in the words. On my right, his arm resting lightly against mine, Gene, my boyfriend of two years, sang in a low, off-key voice. A different sort of harmony. I sang, too, and let the ease of this fellowship, these friendships, calm me. The words of the chorus echoed the shared faith that brought us to this place: "Man shall not live by bread alone, / But by every word / That proceeds out from the mouth of God. / Hallelu, Hallelujah!"

My church youth group was my social center. Even though most of us attended different high schools, my closest friends sat with me here in the Christian Education wing of our sprawling church in Ottawa's downtown. For almost four years, our lives had intertwined during these weekly Wednesday night gatherings, youth activities on weekends, overnight retreats, and Sunday morning worship. Outside of my family, the people in this circle were the ones who knew me best.

The song faded as Chuck palmed the strings of his guitar. He rested the instrument in its black case and said, "As we enter this time of prayer, does anyone have anything they'd like to share?" He picked up a brown, leather notebook and pencil, ready to write down the requests. His smile was an invitation to bank on God's promises. Apprehension crawled up my spine.

No one ever liked being the first to speak, so it took some prompting. "I know that a lot of you have exams coming up," Chuck said. "I'll be praying for clear minds and good studying." Calculus wheels started spinning in my head. Before this advanced class, I'd never struggled with math. Even with private tutoring from a retired math professor in our neighborhood, I was not getting it. Derivatives. Limits. Rates of change. None of it made sense to me. As the midterm approached, I could use all the prayer I could get.

"I have a praise," Kim, a perky ninth grader, said from across the circle. Her face beamed as she held up her right arm. "I got my cast off! Finally!" She'd broken her wrist skating in January and for the last two months had sported a white plaster cast, covered in colorful signatures, many of them ours.

"That's good news!" Chuck said, making a note in his journal. "Anybody else?"

A few others from around the circle chimed in with words of gratitude: the safe return of family members who'd been traveling, the success of our recent youth retreat, praise for the welcome signs of approaching spring.

"My grandmother is having gallbladder surgery on Friday," Cody said running his fingers through his spiked, brown hair. "Pray for a speedy recovery."

The mention of surgery sparked a litany of requests as everyone sifted through their own illness inventories: relatives who were sick, friends and acquaintances in the hospital. As usual, a competition of sorts unfurled. Whose request could beat the last one? Chuck's notebook page was filling up.

"I have a friend at school whose mother was just diagnosed with breast cancer," Lauren said, picking at the chipped pink polish on her thumbnail. "She's having a really tough time, and I don't know how to help her." Her eyes watered as she scanned the group.

"The best thing you can do is be there for her," Chuck said, leaning forward, his elbows resting on his knees, compassion infusing his voice. "Let her know she's not alone, and tell her you are praying for her. God is the greatest comfort you can give to anyone."

Lauren nodded and wiped her nose with the tissue that Carol, one of the other youth leaders, passed her way.

I hugged my arms across my chest and stared down at the steely industrial carpet at my feet. I focused on a dark stain, about an inch in diameter. I'd been trying to hold onto the promise of God's comfort. Hard. I bit my lip. Even though the prayer request burning on my tongue would outdo everything on Chuck's list, I said nothing.

A few days earlier, my parents had come back from a week-long trip to Halifax, where they flew to see my dad's doctors. Dad had been quiet and withdrawn since their return. He fell asleep more often in the evenings than I was used to seeing. Last night, I asked him a question at dinner. When he turned to me and said, "What was that, Mel?" like he was emerging from a thick fog, his eyes taking too long to focus, I felt like I'd just pulled him back from somewhere far away. My mind cycled through the facts my parents had revealed since their return. Lowered T-cell count. A significant drop since December. "Dad is getting sicker," Mom said when I worked up the courage to ask for details about what these changes meant. She looked older somehow as she faced me from across the counter in the kitchen. Her eyes swam with tears and undisguised fear. "We've got some decisions to make."

I did not share this story and ask for prayer, though, as Chuck leaned back and waited for further requests. Despite the closeness I felt to this group, the only person in the room who knew anything about my dad's HIV status, the only person I'd ever told, was Gene. And I wasn't supposed to do even that.

A few months earlier, on his way to drop me off after a movie with friends, Gene had steered his mother's yellow Camaro into the empty parking lot of a strip mall a few miles from his neighborhood. Dark storefronts lined the one-story building that faced the lot. Gene shifted the car to park and pointed to one of the shops. "That's my father's salon," he said. A muscle in his jaw tightened. Gene lived with his mom. I knew his parents were divorced, but he'd never mentioned the circumstances, and I hadn't pried.

"He lives this close to you?" I asked, unable to hide my shock.

He turned in his seat, took my hand, laced his fingers with mine, and rubbed his thumb against the inside of my palm. His voice filled with an emotion I hadn't heard from him before, "Yeah. He and my mom don't really talk. He's weird, and his life has been pretty messed up." He didn't elaborate on that part of the story. I didn't push. "But lately, he's wanted to see me. I stopped in here the other day, and we had coffee. I just don't really know how this is going to work out." He searched my face, looking for my reaction.

"Do you want to see him more?"

"Maybe. But I'm afraid to hurt my mom. She's given me everything." His eyes, thick-lashed and the color of rich soil, met mine.

"Can you talk to her about it?" I knew Gene's mom, who cut my hair, to be funny and hip. She wore trendy clothes, high boots, and held back her long hair with colorful clips. Blue mascara made her eyes pop. In all the conversations we'd ever had about Gene, her adoration for her son, her only child, was obvious. I knew she'd do anything for him.

"I guess. Sometimes I just wish I could have a normal life like everyone else's. It gets lonely. Like I'm the only one with a screwed-up family." The moisture pooling at the corners of his eyes made my own sting.

"I want to tell you something," I said before I thought about it too much. I was cold. Shivering. Gene squeezed my trembling hand. "My dad's sick. He has AIDS."

In a rush of jumbled sentences that I thought might choke me on their way out, I told him everything: my dad's heart attack, his bypass surgery, the infected blood, the secret we'd been keeping from everyone. "No one knows," I ended. Tears streamed down my cheeks.

Gene didn't let go of my hand, and his features softened. "Mel," he said, his voice unsteady, his cheeks wet too.

"Don't say anything," I interrupted. "I just needed someone to know. I needed *you* to know. I wanted you to know you aren't alone."

He leaned across the gearshift and put his arms around me. I inhaled the musky smell of his deodorant and cried into his shoulder. He cried with me. "Neither are you," he whispered against my hair.

I glanced in Gene's direction now. He was focusing intently on Chuck and what he was saying, his head cocked to one side. Since that night in the Camaro, I'd told Gene a little about my struggle to understand how God fit into my situation and how hard I was finding it to believe in the promises we echoed in songs and scripture. He listened. And he didn't judge because he had his own questions.

I looked around at my friends in the youth group prayer circle. What would they say if I told them about my dad? Would they be as supportive as Gene? I wanted to believe they would be. I wanted to trust in their kindness and love. I wanted to believe that these people wouldn't judge my dad, or me.

But I watched the news. I saw reports echoing the words of Jerry Falwell and other church leaders touting AIDS as a plague sent by God to rid the world of sinners. Falwell was a Christian. He and so many other Christians, including many in my church, had made standing against homosexuality a spiritual crusade. If Falwell and other loud evangelical voices wouldn't separate AIDS from their views on homosexuality and muster compassion for those who suffered, how would my friends in this group?

Chuck asked us to bow our heads and close our eyes. "I'll open our prayer time, and then if you feel like praying for any of these requests, just go ahead. I'll close after a few minutes."

I shut my eyes and listened to the cadence of Chuck's voice.

"God, I just want to thank you for this night," he said. "I want to thank you for the fun and fellowship we've shared and for the thoughtful discussions that went on during our small groups. Thank you for each person here. Thank you, God, for being present in this moment and for hearing us when we pray and acting on our requests."

I forced myself to focus on Chuck's words. I tried to ignore the nagging doubts that tapped at my consciousness. The same ones that surfaced in the darkness when I was lying alone in my room begging God for a miracle. Begging God not to take my dad. When all I could repeat was, "Please."

God's not listening, the doubts said.

After a moment, Carol offered a quiet prayer for Cody's grandmother and the doctors who would be performing the surgery.

When she finished, Chuck waited for one of us to pray. To break the ice for others to follow. The seconds dragged on and the space began to feel uncomfortable. Chairs creaked as people shifted their positions. Someone coughed.

Questions built inside me like a scream. What if none of this was real? What if no one was looking out for me? What if I really was all alone?

"Dear God," I said, pushing back the questions. I clicked into autopilot and drew on the familiar language I'd heard and prayed throughout my life. "Thank you for this night. Thank you for surrounding us with your love and comforting us when we hurt. Be with Lauren this week as she ministers to her friend. Help her to feel your presence as she offers her support. Hold her close, God. Amen."

A LIFE DIMINISHED

Viewed from the perspective of suffering, AIDS must rank with smallpox, plague, and leprosy in its capacity to menace and hurt, to burden and spoil human experience, and to elicit questions about the nature of life and its significance.

PAUL FARMER, M.D. AND ARTHUR KLEINMAN, M.D.
"AIDS as Human Suffering," *Daedalus*

Daddy's Girl
2012

On a winter afternoon, Lily skipped ahead of me onto our house's porch through the garage door. She dropped her backpack on the floor, pulled her arms from her jacket, and threw it inside her cubby in a heap, ignoring the hooks on the wall. She kicked off her boots. "You know how we are studying plant cycles, right?" she said, digging through her backpack and pulling out her pink homework binder.

"Mmm hmm," I responded, unzipping my coat and making a deliberate but unnoticed show of hanging it on the hook before walking into the kitchen.

"Well, in this video we watched today, they started talking about how the plant cycle is like the human and animal reproductive cycle. And they showed an egg. And sperm." She paused, her brows furrowed, her wide eyes searching my face, expecting my shock to match hers. "It was really gross. And in-a-ppro-priate." She landed hard on each syllable of the final word.

I stifled a laugh with a cough. Lily was very literal.

A few weeks ago, Chris and I had sat her down with Will to have a conversation about the nuts and bolts of human reproduction. My brother David and his husband, Ian, were expecting a baby through a surrogate. The untraditional conception of this new cousin required explanation. We suspected that, at twelve, Will already possessed some of the knowledge we were going to share. I'd taught middle school. The boys sweated hormones, and their banter was always laced with innuendo. Plus, his seventh-grade health class recently included an "Understanding the Human Body" component. We'd tried to have this conversation with him before, but he held his ground, refusing to let us corner him into any conversations about sex. The last time I'd tried, on a night when Lily was at gymnastics, and Will, Chris, and I were sharing a plate of nachos at a nearby Mexican restaurant, he'd turned to Chris and asked, "Why is she so *obsessed* with this?"

The information about conception and the challenge it posed for same sex couples was new for Lily, though. I'd kept it simple. "So, to make a baby, you need two things: an egg and sperm," I looked to Chris to jump in, but all he did was nod. I shot him my best thanks-for-the-support-and-equal-partnership glare and continued, "The egg comes from a woman and the sperm comes from a man. Obviously, Uncle Dave and Uncle Ian don't have the egg." I explained enough to help Will and Lily understand why their uncles needed some outside assistance to begin their family.

At one point in the conversation, I mentioned that it wouldn't be appropriate for Lily or Will to have this kind of dialogue with their friends because those conversations should be initiated with their own parents. Apparently, encountering a discussion of human eggs and sperm in her fourth-grade science class was a breach of Lily's sense of propriety.

"Honey, it's not gross or embarrassing. It's just the natural process of how life works," I said, still trying not to laugh.

"So, what exactly am I supposed to do about it?" she demanded, her arms crossed, her feet planted on the kitchen's hardwood floor.

Lily's logical mind was never satisfied with pithy responses to her questions, and, for a nine-year-old, she possessed a pretty sharp B.S. detector. "So, what exactly …?" was a regular precursor to a lengthier conversation than I'd planned for.

"You don't have to *do* anything, Lil," I said, pulling up one of the kitchen island's low barstools in front of her. "But you can talk to me about it if you have questions." I said this last part cautiously, knowing that opening the floor for questions meant I'd get them. Challenging ones.

She bit her lip and looked down, her blonde ponytail falling across her shoulder. Her mind searched for a good starting place. She raised her gaze and her face lit.

"What're tampins?" she asked.

"Tampins?"

"You know that book? The one I got from Santa? It talks about tampins."

A light switched on in my own brain. Lily was verging on the brink of puberty. Anticipating her need for answers, "Santa" had included a book called *The Care and Keeping of You* in her Christmas stocking. Published by the American Girl Company, it presented facts about good health and hygiene and, without entering into some of the more complex issues of sexuality, it discussed body changes that preteen girls could expect. Accurate and unnerving cartoon drawings accompanied the explanations of things like developing breasts, hair growth, and preparations for getting your period.

"Oh, *tampons*," I said. "You know how I talked to you about expecting your period in the next few years? Tampons are used for that."

"Okay." She arched her back and executed a back walkover in the open space between the island and the counter, her toes pointed, her legs precise. Movement grounded Lily. It hadn't been a tough decision for us to enroll her in gymnastics when she was five after we realized it would be better for her to be cartwheeling on mats instead of in the aisles of Target. Once upright, she turned back to me. "And when will I start wearing a bra?"

"When you start developing breasts."

"And when exactly will that be?"

I explained that there was no predetermined date, but that sometime between then and when she started middle school she'd probably notice some changes. "You're still pretty small, though, Lil, so it might be a little longer."

"How will I know when to start wearing one?" She twisted her ponytail around her fingers.

"I'll tell you."

She sighed, her relief obvious in her movements. I walked over to the counter and started preparing dinner while Lily leaned against the island and meandered through a series of queries: "And where exactly will I be growing hair?" "What's acne?" "When exactly should I start shaving my legs?" "What are hormones?" "Is my hair greasy?" The conversation spiraled off on funny tangents involving hygiene tips, me filling in the gaps of her knowledge when necessary, not offering more than she needed for the moment.

"What about boys?" she ventured, shifting from one foot to the other.

"What about boys?" I asked, pausing my sautéing of the veggies in the frying pan on the stove, keeping my voice even and alert.

I remembered fourth grade in vivid detail. I remembered sprawling in the newly mown grass of my next-door neighbor's yard one spring evening with Joshua Carter, a boy from down the street. We'd ended up alone after a game of hide and seek with the other neighborhood kids had fizzled out. Dark crept in. Our moms would soon sound the neighborhood call that would send everyone in for the night. The dying light cast shadows on the lawn, further darkening the area where we sat. A strange flutter in my stomach warmed my cheeks, and I felt unexpectedly shy. I felt Joshua's shyness too. We'd been buddies since kindergarten, but something was changing. He reached out a tentative hand, and his fingers wrapped around mine. A current of energy stole up my arm. I didn't pull my hand away.

"Maybe I'll just kiss you?" he said, his tone a lot less bold than his words.

"Okay," I said.

He leaned in and touched his lips to mine for the briefest of instants. The world seemed suddenly bigger than I'd known. I was ten, only a few months older than Lily. I didn't feel ready to navigate the whole relationship path with her just yet. I wanted her to stay little a while longer.

"What about boys?" I repeated, the spatula still poised.

"Well, how exactly will I know who to marry?" she asked. My shoulders relaxed. I switched the burner to low and left the veggies to simmer.

"That's a long way off," I said, turning and wrapping her in my arms. "Just enjoy having lots of friends right now." I kissed the top of her blonde head and smelled the strawberry of her shampoo. "Both boys and girls."

"Couldn't I just marry Daddy?" She persisted, pulling free of my embrace, her hazel eyes earnest.

I laughed. "Not if the police have anything to say about it."

"But it would make everything easy. I love him the best."

It made complete sense to her. Of all the "boys" in her world, Chris ranked at the top. Lily and I had our own unique relationship, but there was no question that she was Daddy's girl. Their bond formed the moment Chris first looked into her eyes and saw his own staring back at him. He was the hub of her existence.

As a little girl, she'd toddled after him, keeping step with Will, vying for Chris's attention with any antic that would generate his laughter. She'd made his passion for New England sports her own, and loved nothing more than curling up next to him on what she referred to as "Daddy's bed," even though I slept there too. She fell asleep to the banter Chris shared with Will between plays of the Bruins, Celtics, Red Sox, or Patriots. From the basketball court, soccer field, or balance beam, her eyes searched the crowd for Chris, flashing a little smile after a basket or goal. She smiled at me, too, but she sought his approval. Though I was sometimes on the outside, I didn't begrudge them their bond.

My dad was my first love too.

Shards of Grief

I WAS ABOUT five minutes early when I parked myself on the gaudy, double wide wingback chair against the wall of Dr. B's waiting room. I tried to focus on the magazine I'd grabbed off the side table. It was a year-old Thanksgiving issue of a *Better Homes and Gardens*. The cover photo of a caramel apple-cherry pie topped with intricate leaf cutouts had caught my eye, but when I flipped to the recipe and saw that it used words like "compote" and required at least ten steps that totaled two hours' worth of preparation, I knew I was out of my league. I tossed the magazine back on the table.

I began, instead, a mental redesign of the waiting room. I was not a fan of the current set up. It was too symmetrical. Two chairs separated by a low, square table rested against the wall opposite me. A fake potted tree pushed into the corner. A half-filled water cooler sat next to it. A metal coat rack stood in the other corner. In my imagined makeover, I'd give it a warmer paint color as an alternative to the dull pinkish-beige currently on the walls, add lamps to replace the overhead fluorescents, and realign the framed bowl-of-fruit painting, bulletin board, and wall calendar. But, my first order of business would be rearranging the furniture.

The space was only about five feet wide from wall to wall, so, on the occasions when clients waited for one of the other therapists in the practice at the same time as I waited for Dr. B, we ended up facing each other, doing the awkward dance of trying to avoid eye contact while we wondered, *Why are you here?*

Simply shifting the two chairs to the other wall so that the seats were kitty-cornered rather than across from each other would make things so much more comfortable. And since I had a stake in the place—it was a year and a half into our work together and my crazy was single-handedly funding Dr. B's retirement—my personal comfort should be a priority.

One of these days, I was going to tell Dr. B my Waiting Room Beautification Plan. Not today, though. Today, I didn't know what I was going to tell him, or whether I could tell him anything at all.

His mother had died the week before. That day was his first day back in the office.

When we'd last met, three weeks earlier, I told Dr. B that even though I'd known for ten years that my father was going to die, nothing had prepared me for what it would feel like to lose him. Dad was the mooring to which I'd attached since I was a little girl. Without him, I felt untethered. No matter how much time passed, I couldn't shed that feeling. "I miss him *all* the time," I said. "He should be here." The lament tumbled from my lips, and the force of my grief hit me hard. I covered my face with my hands while sobs shook my shoulders.

Dr. B knew the moments that weren't meant for words. For what felt like a long time, my sobs were the only sound. I'd cried plenty of times in his office—pretty much every time—but not like this. This crying was raw, every nerve ending exposed. My insides spread wide open for view.

Eventually, I reached for a tissue from the box on the table and wiped my eyes and nose. I looked at him then, poised to apologize for falling apart.

He spoke first, though, and his voice was accepting and gentle. "Tell me what you miss about your dad."

It was the first time anyone had invited me, *carte blanche,* to talk about my dad on my terms. And just like on my first visit to Dr. B, I felt like he wanted to know. That there was safety in his presence to feel what I needed to feel. So, I started, scattered memories mingling with my imaginings of what life now would be like with Dad in it.

"This is what you need," Dr. B said, tilting his head to the side, his eyes thoughtful. "Probably what you've needed for a really long time. You need space to talk about your dad. What you loved. What you lost. What you grieve. What you miss." I nodded. "So, we'll keep doing it," he promised, wrapping up our session. "As long as you need to."

A swell of gratitude rose in me. He wasn't recoiling from my stories or from my sadness. He was sitting right in it and offering to come closer. I walked out the door feeling different. Lighter.

But that was three distant weeks ago. Before he called to let me know he was traveling out of state because his mother was ill and we needed to cancel our next appointment. Before I got a second call from his office manager a few days later to cancel two more appointments because Dr. B's mother had died and he was staying at the family home to get everything in order. How the hell was I supposed to walk into that office today and continue talking about my grief when his was so fresh?

My fingers grazed the edge of the white envelope tucked into the side pocket of my handbag. Rather than a Hallmarky, pre-printed sympathy card, I'd chosen a simple blank one, a photo of a lush, green forest on its front. Dr. B, I knew, was a nature guy. I didn't try to find my own words for what felt wordless, and instead I copied lines from a favorite Wendell Berry poem, "The Peace of Wild Things," inside.

The time I spent agonizing over whether I should give him this card was beyond ridiculous. I wanted to be respectful and appropriate, but the lines of this relationship felt newly hazy to me. "He's not your friend; he's your therapist," I reminded myself. But the previous week, when I'd gotten the call from the office manager, the sadness that blanketed me at the news of his loss felt a lot like what I'd feel for any one of my close friends in the same circumstance.

My body tensed at the sounds of Dr. B's office door opening and his footsteps padding down the short hallway to the waiting room. He poked his head around the corner, gave me his normal smile, and said, "Come on back, Melanie."

I followed him to his office and tried to keep my breathing even. Tried not to cry. It was too early in the session for the crying. I handed him my check as usual, and he sat at his desk to write out my receipt. I positioned myself on the center cushion of the leather couch and while I waited for him to take his seat across from me, I soothed my palms on my thighs in a repetitive pattern. I'd forgotten my cup of tea, and my hands had nothing to do.

Dr. B settled into his chair. I noticed the dull shadows that ringed his eyes, and, though he was his pleasant self, I sensed he was weary. "So," he said, the standard opening for me to share what was on my mind. He wove his fingers together across his bent knee.

There were things I was supposed to say. "I'm so sorry about your mom," I managed haltingly, and my voice cracked at the end. The words felt artificial and cliché.

"Thank you," he said.

"Are you okay?" I didn't know if I was allowed to ask this, we only talked about his personal life if he brought it up in the context of our conversation, but I couldn't help it. I wanted to know.

"I'm okay." His voice remained steady, but there was something in the way he said it that hinted at the sorrow of the past days.

So many other questions sifted through my mind. I wanted to ask about the rest of his family, his siblings, his wife. His two young boys. How were they? Were they okay? I recognized that these weren't my questions to ask. The understood boundaries between us told me that these weren't my answers to know.

"How are you?" He was redirecting.

I looked down at my hands and fiddled with my wedding band, twisting it one way and re-twisting it the other. I felt displaced. Separated from the usual safety of this space. Three weeks ago, I'd felt so at ease that I expressed myself more honestly, exposed my grief more fully, than I ever had before. That ease had vanished. In its place, a giant roadblock of uncertainty detoured my words, made me second-guess what I should and should not say. And, to top things off, I was crying.

"Can you talk to me about what you're feeling?" Dr. B asked.

No, I thought. I can't. That was the whole point. I was surprised at the flash of anger that tied onto these thoughts.

"I don't know how to do this," I choked and swiped in frustration at my tears.

"How to do what?"

"This!" I gestured at him, at myself, at the space between us. "How can I talk to you about my sadness? My pain? It's so selfish." My voice got smaller. "Your mother just died."

"I wondered if this might happen," he said and scratched at his beard. "You feel like you should be taking care of me, right?"

I bit my lip, dropped my eyes, and nodded.

Why shouldn't I? Despite a rational piece of me that knew the parameters of this therapist-client relationship, an emotional piece of me needed the illusion of him as friend. That illusion is what let me open up to him. When my friends were hurting, my instinct was to take care of them.

"Your pattern is to push your own pain aside and focus instead on what you think the people around you need," Dr. B said. Even after our year and a half of work, it was unsettling that he had me pegged so well. He paused, and I listened to the drone of passing cars traveling up and down Amherst Street. The murmur of voices floated through the wall from the office next door.

"I'm not saying it's a bad thing," he said, and paused again before asking gently, "But if you're doing all that caretaking, then who takes care of you?"

A fresh collection of tears filled my eyes.

"I want you to know that I am so grateful for your compassion, Melanie," he said, and bent forward, resting his elbows on his knees. "But I want you to listen to me, to really hear me." His look was pointed, his voice serious. "You don't have to take care of me." He slowed his speech on this last sentence, giving each word equal emphasis. "You don't have to protect me from your pain because you think it might make me sad. My story is not your story. Your story is unique. And I want you to talk about it. You need to talk about it. I'm here to listen."

I felt like I should launch a protest, but the clamber of emotion inside me wanted to cling to what he was saying and find calm.

"There will be times when our stories intersect, and I'll be feeling some of what you are feeling. That's only natural," Dr. B said. "There's some comfort in those intersections, don't you think?"

"Yes," I whispered and looked over his shoulder out the window where the tall pines across the street swayed to the rhythm of the wind.

"This is me giving you permission to talk about your pain. About your sadness. I'm telling you it's okay."

There was that *carte blanche* invitation again, its sincerity almost painful. My guarded memories, fully formed scenes of a beloved life now disappeared, tugged against their restraints. The roadblock started to crumble. My tension released.

Dr. B leaned in and said, "So, tell me more about your father."

He Was My Favorite

WHEN I SIT down to write a simple description of my dad, I get stuck.
The words I scatter into my sentences in my efforts to give him definition—*brilliant, wise, confident, funny, loving, hardworking, compassionate,
generous, proud, respected, guarded, complicated*—feel stiff and distancing.
In my mind, my dad lives as a medley of images and captured moments
that order and reorder themselves to shape, as best they can, some of
the contours of the man he was. In no particular order, here are some
highlights.

Dad didn't like his coffee too hot. No matter where we were, he'd
scoop an ice cube from his water glass and stir it into his steaming cup
until it dissolved in the dark liquid before taking his first sip.

He could tie a fly onto a fishing line with one hand.

He'd take naps on the family room couch with his glasses still propped
on his face.

He had a secret nickname for almost everyone—comical, often unflat-
tering and bordering on offensive, and inevitably spot on—that would
end up sticking for good. When Mark brought his first girlfriend home
from college, Dad christened her "The Pickle" because that's where she
ranked on his scale of sweetness.

On many nights when he was on call at the hospital, he'd rush home,
still wearing his green scrubs, to sit down with us for a family dinner.
Sometimes he'd be late, and other times he'd be there only a few
minutes before his beeper would sound, beckoning him for a surgical
consult. But he always did his best to show up.

Canned peas on toast—a combination that still makes my stomach
turn—were his comfort food.

He hated his name, and, when he knew he was dying, discharging his characteristic humor, he made my brothers and me promise that we wouldn't get all sentimental and name any of our children Orville in homage to him.

He twiddled his thumbs when he was bored and often made a point of showing me that he was doing it, letting me know that it was okay for me to be bored too.

When I still had my baby teeth, he'd take the first bite of my apple to break the skin for me.

He had a way of buoying my confidence with his.

He was known to press the test button on his hospital pager as an excuse to get up and leave when the sermon at church got too long.

He loved white cake with jam filling and butter icing.

It was his fault we never got perfect attendance in Sunday school because, on those Sunday mornings when the sun's early sparkle promised a beautiful day, a drive to the beach or a hike in the woods often felt like a better option to him than filing into a church pew.

Once, after his diagnosis, he watched a mosquito bite his arm and turned to me with a wry smile and slowly said, "Joke's on the mosquito."

He scratched the inside of his ears with his car keys.

His hands were large and strong and steady.

He liked my hair short, and when I was eleven, he bribed me to cut off the uneven layers I was trying to grow out by letting me get my ears pierced.

He had a deep crease between his eyebrows from years of intense concentration in the operating room.

The first time he gave me a driving lesson, he made me cry before we'd even left the driveway because he got so frustrated when I couldn't master idling in first gear on a hill.

The deepest expression of his faith could be found in his music. He was a gifted pianist and played with the ease of someone speaking his first language. He'd come home from a long day at the hospital and sometimes play for an hour or more straight, transitioning seamlessly from one piece to the next without ever looking at a sheet of music. The stored notes from his memory flowed through his fingers like a prayer.

He despised the Christmas carol, "Little Drummer Boy."

At my brother Michael's wedding, he modeled his thank-you speech to Yvonne's parents after a Baptist three-point sermon, saying simply: "Thanks for the day, thanks for the dinner, thanks for the daughter."

He adored my mother and never let a day go by without letting her, and us, know it.

When we were little, he could stop my brothers and me mid-fight just by taking the wooden spoon out of the kitchen drawer and laying it on the counter.

He taught me how to dive off the diving board by singing the title song to the musical *Oklahoma* exhorting me to hit the water by the time he got to the final "A" when the lyrics spelled out the state name.

He was a gifted speaker with a natural ability to make people pay attention, but on matters of the heart, he was often silent.

On Valentine's Day, he'd bring home a rose for Mom and a rose for me.

He used to call cocktail onions "roly poly onions."

He sent me a letter soon after I'd left for college telling me that things were going downhill in my absence, and that as a result of Mom's new diet, he and David were starving.

He'd nestle me close on the piano bench when I was little, my feet dangling above the floor, and let me rest my hands on top of his while he played.

His sense of humor was quick and dry and irreverent, and he could make me laugh harder than anyone else.

When I called from New Hampshire to tell my parents that Chris and I were engaged, he didn't speak at all and when my mom said, "Orv, say something nice," he got so mad that she called him out, he hung up the phone.

He was never afraid to make his opinion known. Once on an outing with my grandmother, he grabbed a hat that he loathed right off her head and threw it out the car window.

He was a nature guy and found solace in fresh air, the stillness of a fishing stream, a sail on open water, a walk among the trees.

He once wrestled our dog to the floor to pry a chicken bone from between his teeth.

When I was four, he taught me to downhill ski by standing me between his legs and letting me glide down the slope holding on to his knees.

In restaurants, he'd challenge me to lemon sucking contests, each of us shoving a wedge between our teeth and trying to keep a straight face.

He grounded me from church youth group when I was failing calculus my senior year of high school.

He was the surgeon on call, charged with being at the ready at the hospital, for the visits to Moncton in 1984 of both Pope John Paul II and Queen Elizabeth II.

In my first month of college, he stayed on the phone with me for over two hours to help me understand the American two-party system so I could write a paper for my political science class.

His approval meant everything to me.

He disapproved of all my boyfriends.

When we'd take long family road trips, he'd come out of the gas station with a brown paper bag full of mystery items (chocolate bars, bags of chips, cans of soda) and offer each one for auction to the highest bidder from the back seat, without telling us the other options.

He approached purchasing a car with the precision of a nuclear scientist, meticulously researching his options, weighing the pros and cons of the features and specs, and determining a price threshold before ever setting foot on the lot.

He was a man of abiding faith and wrestled with deep doubts. He said to me once, "I don't think I'd be a Christian if I thought Christians were what Christianity was all about."

On Christmas morning, he always made a glass of fresh-squeezed orange juice just for me.

He wore the same tan Tilley hat every time we went sailing.

He'd latch onto movie lines and turn them into family mantras. A few of his favorites–from *The Color Purple*: "It's gonna rain on yo' head;"

from *Trading Places:* "Looking good, Billy Ray!" "Feeling Good, Lewis!"; from *The Russians are Coming! The Russians are Coming!:* "Emergency! Everybody to get from street!"

When he got sick, he founded his own private "don't sweat the small stuff" club called WGAS (Who Gives a Shit) and let me become an honorary member.

He was a skilled negotiator and loved the challenge of haggling with salespeople to get the best deal.

On my wedding day, while we stood at the back of the chapel waiting for our cue, he whispered this effort to calm my nerves: "It's not too late. One word and we're out of here."

He wouldn't hesitate to get up and file us all out of a restaurant after we'd been seated if it didn't meet his expectations.

He could write limericks on the fly.

When we were little and the hour-long drive to our cottage felt endless, he'd make up stories about "The Ghost of the McLaughlin Road" named for the longest section of the trip.

One of his favorite expressions was, "Lighten up, fella."

He had zero tolerance for pretension.

When his mind was made up, it was rare that anyone could change it.

He always expected us to perform—singing or playing our musical instruments— when we had company.

He scared me a little bit.

He played the guitar, so there was always singing around the fire on camping trips.

He set expectations for us that were almost impossible to meet.

When Bailey had to be put to sleep while I was away at my last year of college, he called me afterwards and said, "If I had my choice, I think that's how I'd like to go too."

He knew pretty much everything about everything.

We all understood he was the guy in charge and his way was the one and only way.

—

Dad was born in the little town of Windsor, Nova Scotia in 1942. Just months before Dad's birth, when World War II broke out, my grandfather felt the press of a deep sense of duty to help protect the country he'd left as a young man, and he enlisted in the Royal Canadian Army without telling my grandmother. He just showed up at the house one day in full military uniform. I learned only recently this piece of my grandparents' history. The summer my grandfather enlisted, they'd brought their three daughters to Kennetcook, Nova Scotia, for a holiday with my grandmother's parents. I don't have firsthand specifics of this event, but my imagination fills them in. I picture Grammie standing at the sink in the kitchen, rinsing dishes in soapy water. The afternoon sun warms her face as it streams through the open window. She looks out at the lush green of the wild blueberry fields in the distance. A tall man in military dress strides along the walkway toward the house, his arms swinging loosely at his sides. It takes her a minute to recognize her husband. This man wearing the signature khaki uniform of the Royal Canadian Armed Forces is her husband. She grips the sink and doubles over, a wave of nausea throwing her off balance. Something inside her breaks. That something stayed broken. Because he'd died before I was born, I'd never known my grandfather. My grandmother, though, was a part of my life growing up, and she lived with us for three years when I was a preteen. She was not an easy woman. She was rigid in her rules and quick to criticize. Even though she was in her early seventies when she lived with us, she seemed to me like a very old woman. I remember how she'd shuffle up the stairs each morning, a comb stuck in the back of her hair, and sit down at the kitchen table: an unspoken message for my mother to fix her up. The added details about my grandfather's enlistment make me wonder now about her hard-edged exterior. About the unhappiness that I sensed in her.

My grandfather served overseas for the first four years of Dad's life, seeing him for the first time when he was two years old. As a military chaplain, my grandfather ministered to wounded and dying soldiers and one of his main duties was conducting funeral services for fallen Canadian servicemen. More than once, he buried a hundred soldiers in a day. As was the case for so many others, the trauma of war had a profound effect on him and he did not return the same man he'd been when he left. On the day he arrived home, he walked down the ship's gangplank, smoking a cigarette. My grandmother turned away from him, got in the car, and refused to get out. In her sheltered, fundamentalist Christian upbringing, cigarettes, alcohol, and playing cards were equally taboo. To her, my grandfather's new dependency was a sin. They would not talk about the unimaginable things he'd experienced. He would carry their weight on his own, and a gulf of words unsaid would exist between them. My father grew up learning this way of keeping silent about the hard stuff, and by watching him, we learned it too.

Not long after the war ended, my grandparents settled in Moncton, New Brunswick, where my grandfather served as a Baptist minister, and this was where Dad spent most of his childhood and adolescence. They lived in a modest home and money was tight. Despite the financial obstacles, his parents nurtured in him and his three older sisters a drive to achieve, and my father did not disappoint. He was equally gifted as a musician and an intellect. He studied classical piano and excelled in school. When Dad was in grade two, Grammie, who'd been a schoolteacher in a one-room rural schoolhouse before she'd married my grandfather, marched in and declared that my father was too smart for what they were studying and needed a bigger challenge. He moved up that year to grade three. In high school, when given the chance to do two years of study in one year, he took it. He was only fifteen when he graduated from high school. The prestigious Governor General's Medal he won that year for the highest grade point average sits on a shelf in my bedroom, a keepsake my mother gave me after Dad died. He received a full-ride scholarship to McGill University and began his studies in the fall of 1958 toward a Bachelor of Science degree on the path to fulfill his lifelong dream of being a doctor.

I wonder sometimes what my childhood might have been like if the script for how to achieve a successful life hadn't been written into Dad's life so early. Would the intensity of his own ambitions have been less overt in the way he parented us? When I was growing up, would there still have been positioned the ever-raising, elusive bar of excellence as the only standard for me and for my three brothers?

In Dad's third year of university, his father died. My grandfather's health had deteriorated after he'd returned from the war, and though his doctors always treated it as heart disease, after his own training in cardiac and thoracic surgery, Dad would later decide that it was more likely his father had suffered from pulmonary disease and, probably, lung cancer. Dad was just seventeen when his father died, though, and the loss crushed him. He couldn't focus, and the added pressure to maintain the demanded grade point average of his scholarship over-whelmed him. For the first time in his academic career, his grades faltered and he lost his scholarship. He might not have completed his degree if not for the generosity of family friends and the savings he'd accumulated during high school and college summers cleaning used cars at a dealership and delivering newspapers for miles. He graduated with his bachelor's in science and was accepted to McGill's prestigious medical school.

My father met my mother when they were both fourteen. My mother had just moved to town and started attending the same high school. Her father was an executive vice president for the Canadian National Railway and she spent her childhood and adolescence moving between Montreal, Winnipeg, and Moncton—main hubs for the railroad. Unlike my father, my mother grew up surrounded by wealth. She lived in a spacious home in downtown Moncton where her parents enter-tained railway officials and local friends regularly. Despite this differ-ence in my parents' backgrounds, they shared a deep Christian faith and love for music, and the foundation of their friendship remained strong even after my father left for McGill.

Two years after my father started there, my mother also studied at McGill, earning a bachelor's degree in critical care nursing while

Dad was working on his MD. They married immediately after my father graduated from medical school and started their life together in Montreal. During his two-year family medicine internship at Montreal General Hospital, Dad was given the opportunity to do extensive clinical work in surgery and developed a passion for the specialty. After finishing his internship, though, he and my mother moved back to Moncton, where my father took over a busy family practice from a retiring doctor, and he worked as a general practitioner for five years so they could begin their family and gain some financial grounding. Dad had watched his parents' lifelong struggle to make ends meet, and he was determined to provide a more stable environment for his own family.

Dad's early years as a family practitioner in Moncton earned him a reputation as a skilled and compassionate doctor with a deeply kind bedside manner that distinguished him throughout his whole medical career. "Are you Dr. Messenger's daughter?" strangers would ask me throughout my childhood once they heard my name. Their voices soaked with admiration, they'd then launch into some version of the same story: Dad had figured out their (or their spouse's, parent's, child's, sibling's, aunt's, uncle's) mystery illness, given them a diagnosis, and saved their life. Whether the stories were exaggerated for effect or not, I didn't know. What I did know was that being Melanie Messenger, Dr. Messenger's daughter, made me important.

Only a few months after I was born, Dad left his family practice, and we moved to Toronto, where he began an intensive surgical residency at the University of Toronto. My mother stayed home with three children under the age of three while Dad worked a grueling twenty-four hours on, twenty-four hours off call schedule, sleeping every other night at the hospital. After three years in Toronto, we lived for a year in Texas where Dad studied cardiac surgery at Baylor University Hospital in Dallas. He was part of the first group of doctors in Canada to become a fellow in the new specialty of general thoracic surgery, treating and operating on diseases of the chest wall, lungs, esophagus, diaphragm, and mediastinum. Equipped with this expertise, he returned to Moncton and built a thriving surgical practice, serving as the only thoracic surgeon in the Canadian Maritimes and was eventually named chief of surgery at Moncton Hospital. The bedside manner he'd learned as a family doctor and maintained in this new role made him a surgeon who challenged the notions of arrogance and abrasiveness that often define those who pursue surgery. After Dad died, my mother received hundreds of handwritten notes of sympathy, many of them from his former colleagues, his patients, and their families. Again and again, they spoke to his compassion, his way of listening, his generosity of time, and his genuine care.

We eventually moved into a modern and expansive split-level house with high, sloping ceilings that sat on a hill overlooking the city on a large piece of property with an in-ground pool and woods on three sides. Each bedroom had a private balcony, and my grandmother lived in a large downstairs suite. Until I was thirteen, I lived an idyllic, privileged life. Mom and Dad had a loving marriage and dedicated themselves to creating a happy home. Our lives were busy and filled with swimming lessons and music recitals, church on Sundays, family ski trips in the winter, and summer days at our secluded cottage on a coastal river in Kent County, New Brunswick.

Then one day, Dad finished a lengthy surgery, stepped out of the operating room, and collapsed, and what I'd always believed to be unbreakable shattered.

Who He Was Before
1976

WHEN I WAS four years old, I crashed headfirst into a metal staircase in our apartment courtyard because I was so busy trying to tag Tommy Adler that I forgot to duck. The impact threw me off my feet and sent me flying backward into the grass. I was crying by the time I sat back up, and Tommy was gone. When I reached my fingers to the throbbing spot on my forehead and felt something wet, I cried harder. The blood stung my eyes, and mixing with my tears, started gushing down my face and dripping onto my yellow tank top.

"Hey, are you okay?" The voice belonged to the paperboy, a lanky teenager who lived a few doors down from us. His canvas bag, heavy with newspapers, was slung across his lean shoulders. I was wailing now. I couldn't find my voice. He helped me to my feet and told me to keep my hand on my forehead. He took my other hand in his and guided me around the side of the building and down the sidewalk to the front entrance of our unit. I was too busy focusing on the blood still dripping onto my shirt to care that this boy I hardly knew was holding my hand.

Mom answered the door on the first knock, probably already on her way to find me because I hadn't run past the back patio slider where she monitored my play from the kitchen. Her eyes widened when she saw my tear-streaked, bloody face. She pulled me to her and cried, "Oh, Melanie! What happened?"

"I … hit … my … head," I managed to wedge the words into the spaces between my sobs.

111

"I'd say so," Mom said. She thanked my rescuer, sent him back to his paper route, and carried me into the kitchen. She sat me on the laminate counter by the sink and gave me a flowered dishtowel to press against my forehead while she wet a facecloth under the faucet. She wiped the blood off my face and hands. "Now, let's take a closer look," she said and gently lifted the towel. I watched the deepening crease between her eyebrows while she examined the wound, pushing and pulling the surrounding skin. My head still throbbed, but I managed to stop crying. I was letting Mom's reactions determine whether or not I'd launch into a new wave of tears.

"Well," she said. "It looks like we get to go visit Daddy."

A thrill of excitement surged through me and drowned out some of my fear. The hospital! I didn't remember ever having to be taken to the hospital before.

I watched Mom lift the telephone receiver from its cradle on the wall, put it to her ear, and dial a number on the round dial. She twisted the long cord around her fingertips. "Yes," she said when someone picked up on the other end, "This is Dr. Messenger's wife. Can you please page him and tell him I'm on my way to the emergency room with our daughter? She's going to need stitches in her forehead, and I'd like him to meet us there." She paused. "Thank you so much." She pushed down the metal cradle, but kept the receiver pressed against her ear while she spun another number. This time, she called the house where my older brothers were playing down the street and asked the mother to keep them there until we came home.

"What are stitches?" I asked when I was settled in the back seat of our station wagon, a fresh t-shirt and a clean tea towel replacing the bloodied ones. The air-conditioner blasted cold air from the front, and goose bumps prickled the skin on my bare legs.

"They are little threads that help to keep your skin closed when a cut is deep like the one you have," she said. "Like sewing."

"Do they hurt?" My lip started to tremble again as the image of a sewing needle worried its way into my head.

"You won't feel anything because they'll freeze the skin around your cut." I tried to picture how that would work, imagining special ice that they might use, as Mom turned into the driveway of the hospital. I'd been here before to see where Dad worked, and sometimes, when I was not in school, I'd go with Mom to drop him off on these days when she needed the car. We looped around the driveway in front of the towering building and followed the sign that began with the letter E, "for Emergency," Mom said. She parked the station wagon, came around to open my door, and cautioned: "Keep the towel pressed to your head." We walked hand-in-hand toward the wide glass doors under the awning with big, red letters that spelled the same thing as the sign on the road.

"Emergency," I said out loud, storing the word in my memory.

The doors slid open with a *whoosh* before we even stepped onto the mat, and there was Daddy. He was dressed in green surgical scrubs and a white lab coat. He bent down and scooped me into his arms. "What happened to you, Meligans?"

I wrapped my legs around his waist and played with the stethoscope at his neck. "I crashed into the stairs in the backyard," I said. I loved to be carried. I'd look down from my special perch at my brothers, too big now to be held, and relish this one thing that I could do that they couldn't.

"Let me see," he said. I moved the towel away from my forehead. He touched the edges of the cut, his large, capable hands gentle against my skin. It hurt only a little bit. He pressed the towel back in place, grinned at me, adjusting his thick-rimmed glasses and said, "We'll get you fixed up in no time." He balanced me with one arm and put his other hand on Mom's back, steering her through the double doors. He was in charge now. This was his hospital. The place he did the important work of making people better when they were sick or hurt. As he carried me down the hallway, bypassing the crowded waiting area, and paused at the long admissions desk to ask the nurse which exam room was ready for us, I felt important too.

We entered a square room with open doorways along the outside wall that led into smaller rooms. Nurses and other doctors in the same scrubs Dad was wearing sat behind a tall counter. "Who do we have here, Dr. Messenger?" A nurse with curly brown hair asked as we approached.

"This is my daughter, Melanie, and my wife, Dorothy," Dad said. "It looks like Little Mel is going to definitely need some stitches," he added.

"Well, aren't you a lucky girl," the nurse said. "We just happen to have the best stitcher waiting for you." She pointed to the man sitting beside her. "Dr. Davison here came down on special request from your dad." She leaned in close, like she was telling me a secret. "He only stitches up the extra special patients."

The other doctor stood. He was almost as tall as my dad. He flashed me a smile and winked. "I promise to be gentle," he said, "but just in case, we'll bring Cindy here along to help. And I guess your dad and mom can come too. Does that sound all right to you?" I nodded. I didn't know if I should be scared or excited as Dad carried me into an exam room. Mom followed closely behind.

The whole thing was fast. It turned out the freezing was not any sort of ice, but I was so enthralled by the blood pressure cuff and pump that Dad let me play with, I hardly noticed the big needle that delivered the anesthetic. And then, my whole forehead got tingly, and I only felt a bit of pressure when Dr. Davison sewed up my cut. "You're a pretty strong girl," he said when he was finished. "Five stitches and not a peep. I've stitched up plenty of grownups who don't behave that well." A current of pleasure ran through me, and when I looked at my dad, I could tell by his smile that he was proud.

"Do you want to see?" Dad asked and held a mirror in front of me. He brushed aside my bangs, and I saw a big, purple bump on my forehead, and, in the center, a neat line of black, knotted threads. They looked sort of scary and a bit gross. But there was something about them that made me feel special too. I reached up, about to touch them, but Dad stopped me with a warning about scarring and infections.

I put my hand down and turned to Mom. "Wait 'til Michael and Mark see this!" My older brothers were not easy to impress, but I was convinced these stitches would do the trick.

"You tell those brothers of yours that I said you were my bravest patient today," Dr. Davison said and gave me a high five. He shook my dad's hand, saying something about being "on-call if there are any problems" before he headed out the door.

"I think that somebody deserves a treat after all of this, don't you think, Dorsie?" Dad said as he lifted me off the bed.

"I think so," Mom said and reached for my hand. Dad led us back out past the nurses' station. The nurse, Cindy, gave me a little wave, and another nurse smiled and greeted my dad. Everybody knew him. My sandals slapped against the linoleum as we walked down another hallway.

We turned into a small corridor, and Dad pointed to a gray vending machine against the wall and said, "I bet you'll find something you like in there." While Mom dug in her purse for two quarters, he read me the names of the different candy held by metal coils behind the glass: "KitKats, Mars, M&Ms, Reese's Peanut Butter Cups, Three Musketeers. . ."

"That one," I said as soon as I heard him read the last words. That's what Dad called Michael, Mark, and me: his three musketeers. I didn't know there was a candy bar. I wondered if Michael and Mark knew. Something else I'd get to tell them.

The twisting coil dropped the silver package from its perch after I fed the coins into the slot and Dad pushed the buttons. I reached into the opening at the bottom, folded my fingers around the bar, and pulled it out. I ripped open the wrapper and bit into the thick, delicious rectangle of fluffy nougat cream coated with chocolate.

"Good?" Dad asked, leading us over to a bench against the wall. I nodded. I relaxed against its back, snuggled between my parents. I was starting to feel sleepy.

A series of shrill beeps interrupted the quiet and made me jump. Dad reached into his pocket for his pager and pushed the button to stop the beeping. "Back to work for me," he said. He turned to Mom. "I'll walk you out first."

We made our way back down the hallway and through a doorway that returned us to the emergency room waiting area. Dad's beeper went off again when we got to the entrance. He bent down and planted a kiss on the top of my head, gave Mom a peck on the cheek, and said, "I'll see you later on." I watched him walk back past the waiting room and stand behind the big desk to talk on the telephone. I wondered who was on the other end. Maybe somebody else needed stitches. Or an operation. Dad did those too.

Mom and I walked through the sliding doors and into the afternoon heat. I looked back as they began to close behind us and saw Dad disappear through another doorway. I squared my shoulders and kept walking, secure in the knowledge that no matter whom he was going to see now, when he came home later, he'd be focused on taking care of me.

Who He Became After
1987

TO CAP OFF an extended weekend excursion to my aunt and uncle's in Montreal, my family, sans Michael away at school, was headed to an Expos game. My first visit to a major league ballpark. August sun warmed the air, but the slant of the light signaled the approach of fall. We walked along the bustling sidewalk, swept up in the excited momentum of the game day throng going to Olympic Stadium. Built for the 1976 Summer Games, the stadium's expansive dome stretched out ahead of us like a UFO landed in the middle of the city. We paused at a curb, the orange hand of the pedestrian signal delivering its message not to walk.

The street before us teemed with midday traffic. Montreal was metropolitan and multicultural. Cars carried men and women of different colors and ethnicities. I was still acclimating to the diversity we'd encountered since our move to this part of Canada at the beginning of the year. My childhood in Moncton, New Brunswick, a quiet city at the center of the Canadian Maritimes, had not offered such exposure.

"Stop, Mark," David said for the umpteenth time since we'd parked the car a few blocks away. Mark kept tipping the rim of David's newly purchased Expos cap back each time he tried to straighten it over his brow. David was laughing, though, enjoying the attention from his older brother. I stood next to Mom and Dad, shielding myself from being pulled into my brothers' teasing. I was happy for this change of pace and setting. Being here had relaxed some of the strain and uncertainty that defined our new life in Ottawa. It had been a good break for all of us.

"The retractable roof on the dome was supposed to be the first of its kind and ready for the Olympics," Dad said, pointing across the street. "When they couldn't get it to work, there were a lot of unhappy Canadians."

I half-listened to his tour-guide monologue, more interested in the rumblings of my stomach telling me it was almost lunchtime and wondering what kind of food they had at the ballpark.

A flash of red passed to my right. A boy ran into the street, a brown grocery bag in his arms. There was no time to react. A maroon sedan struck him, the force jettisoning his body in the air. He hung there, a rag doll with a look of surprise frozen on his face. He crashed back down on the car's hood and shattered the windshield. The sound exploded in the silent paralysis of the instant. He landed a few feet away on the pavement with a stomach-turning thud. He lay unmoving, his limbs splayed at impossible angles. The contents of the grocery bag he'd carried scattered, rogue apples rolling across the black asphalt.

Time restarted. People shouted for help, French and English merged in a twisted language of panic. The traffic halted, and drivers exited their vehicles to join the gathering crowd. Terror was engraved on the face of the woman in the sedan. She gripped the steering wheel and started to drive away. A man jumped in front of her car, pounding on the hood. "Stop," he shouted, blocking her advance.

"Someone call an ambulance!" my mom, a registered nurse, yelled and rushed to the boy's side, the first to reach him. Mark was close behind.

I knew I was supposed to follow, but I was rooted in place by confusion. I wanted to rewind the film and excise the footage from my brain. I glanced in the other direction; Dad and David were not in view. My mom motioned me forward. Sirens screamed in the distance. I willed myself to step closer. The boy was conscious. His blond hair fell across his forehead. He might have been eleven or twelve. His eyes were wide open and puzzled. He searched my face for an explanation. A trickle of blood trailed from his mouth down his chin. My mom urged the people who were gathering to keep their distance, instructing Mark to help.

"Talk to him in French, Melanie," she commanded me. I had been in a French-immersion program in school since I started grade one. Now in my first year of high school, I was working to graduate with my bilingual certificate. But I rarely spoke French outside of class.

"Il sera bien. Tu sera bien." It'll be okay. You'll be okay. My French faltered, as though ready to call the bluff of my words. I knew this boy was hurt badly. He tried to speak, but the only sounds he made were rasping breaths, followed by a guttural moan. The sirens grew louder. The boy's eyes began to glaze, no longer focusing on me, or my halting words. I didn't think he heard my stumbling attempts at comfort, but I kept speaking anyway. "Tu sera bien. Tu sera bien. Tu sera bien."

"Where's Dad?" Mom asked, her question steeped in desperation. I knew what she was thinking. My dad could help. He knew what to do. He should be there. But she hadn't seen what I had when the boy crashed down on the car and landed on the street and everyone else crowded toward his unmoving body.

What I saw was my father: the master physician, the proclaimed healer, the trained trauma surgeon; I saw my father, his eyes wild at the sight of the boy getting hit, clamp his hands over his ears and run in the opposite direction as a strangled, animal wail escaped his mouth.

Later, after the paramedics came, steered us aside, and worked frantically over the boy, eventually lifting his motionless body onto a backboard and driving the ambulance away slowly, lights flashing, but no siren, my mother, Mark, and I walked back down the street we'd started on to regroup. A few blocks away, we reunited with David and Dad.

Dad leaned against a telephone pole, his shaking hand clutched to his chest. His face was pale, and worry lines etched his forehead, a dullness shading his eyes. It hurt me to look at him in this defeated state. "I felt like I was having a heart attack," he said in explanation before any of us spoke. It was the only excuse he gave for his retreat. The color drained from my mother's face at his words, but he reassured us that he was feeling better. He asked few questions about the boy. We did not press him with questions of our own.

In the strange way that life resets after moments like this, we retraced our route back to the stadium and attended the game. We cheered for the home team and ate hot dogs and popcorn. We didn't talk about the accident, but I couldn't stop thinking about the boy. Was he dead? What made him run out into the middle of a busy street? Where was he going?

I would not forget the surprised look on the boy's face as his body flew into the air after the car's impact. More often, though, I'd replay my dad's incomprehensible flight; his extended wail, saturated with so much unspoken trauma.

An Uncertain Journey

THE PLIGHT OF the Okies was bringing me down.

The term paper hung over my head. The final project for my senior English class, and I couldn't bear to think about the Joads, their endless trek into the unknown to escape the Dust Bowl, their hopeless future, their ongoing sorrow and loss. John Steinbeck was not an upbeat guy. I briefly wondered if that could be an acceptable thesis for this essay as I stared helplessly at the empty page of my spiral notebook.

The desk lamp, the only light on in my bedroom, cast a dimness across the partially packed boxes that lined the floor. Piles of folded clothes, emptied from my dresser and closet, sat next to them. Earlier, I'd sorted what would get packed away and travel with the movers to Nova Scotia and what I'd keep with me in Ottawa for the summer. The walls were now bare, my framed Monet of the *Woman with the Parasol* and my beloved *Anne of Green Gables* watercolor wrapped and stacked with the other photos and paintings from the rest of the house. My bulletin board still hung above my desk, but the collage of snapshots of friends and family, and mementos including stubs of movie tickets and the dried corsage from my grad dance no longer filled the cork-board. A few stray thumbtacks jutted from its surface. The bookshelf was empty, save for the remaining schoolbooks I needed to finish my finals.

I would graduate from high school in a few days. The next week, Mom, Dad, and David would head cross-country to Nova Scotia and to a new house I'd never seen. Mark would spend the summer on the Georgian Bay working search and rescue for the Coast Guard before beginning medical school at the University of Western Ontario. Michael, just graduated from college, would begin a job in Toronto, as a public policy officer with World Vision Canada, an international relief organization. The decision to move was made after I'd lined up a summer job in the mailroom at the Canadian Medical Protective Association, Dad's firm. It paid far better than anything I might find in Halifax, so we'd decided I should stay and live with my best friend Sherri's family for the summer. I would spend the first two weeks of August in Halifax before leaving for college in Massachusetts.

My family was beginning yet another trek into the unknown. In March, Mom and Dad traveled to Nova Scotia at the recommendation of Dad's cardiologist there to see an infectious disease specialist. Dad's status had changed. HIV no longer lay dormant in the blood cells of his body. The virus was now actively deteriorating his immune system and bringing his T-cell count dangerously low. He was no longer classified as HIV positive. Dad had full-blown AIDS.

This was what we'd all feared. When they'd heard the news, my parents spiraled into a series of rapid decisions: Dad was going to try an experimental drug called AZT. They were moving to Halifax to be close to the infectious disease doctor facilitating that trial. Mom quit her nursing job. With great hesitation, Dad divulged his health status to his boss, one of the few people he'd ever told outside of our family. His boss responded with unexpected compassion and negotiated an arrangement for Dad to continue working for CMPA in one of their remote law offices in Halifax as long as he felt well enough.

Everything had happened so fast. There wasn't a lot of talk about what all these changes meant, and only after the decisions were made did I find out about most of them. But the truth was, apprehension had become a living force in my body, leaving each cell raw. Having to read depressing stories of displaced families wasn't helping.

Dad knocked lightly and peeked into the room. I was surprised he was still up. More and more lately, fatigue sent him to bed early. "How's it going?" he asked.

I was a good student and self-motivated. Excluding a lone calculus debacle the prior semester that led to private tutoring, suspension of all social activities, a barely passing grade, and my dad's final, resigned declaration of "I guess you just don't have that kind of abstract brain," I'd achieved high honors in all of my schoolwork. I'd plugged away and made it through the exams and papers of the past week without much need for intervention. It was just about getting through. Mom and Dad were busy with the burden of the move and worries about his declining health. I didn't want to add to that burden. I tried to muster my characteristic cheerfulness in reply to Dad's question.

I couldn't.

I looked at my dear dad standing in the doorway of my cleared-out bedroom. In his dulled eyes, I could see the strain of all that was happening. A deep yearning rose in me. I wanted him to be okay. I wanted us all to be okay.

I knew we wouldn't be.

"I'm having a hard time ..." I said, surprising myself with my honesty, and my voice trailed off. It wasn't just the paper. It wasn't just graduation. It wasn't just the move. It wasn't just Dad's illness. It was everything. It was the events of the past snarling with the events of the future, sitting on my shoulders, crushing me.

Dad stepped into the room and sat on the edge of my bed and rested his elbows on his knees, his chin leaning on his palms. He didn't speak right away, and I wondered what he was thinking, what encouraging speech he was preparing.

"I know," he said. His words were only a little louder than a whisper.

The standard script had changed. He knew, I thought. For right then, we were not pretending all was well. I didn't have to explain that writing this paper about a family in turmoil felt like writing about our family. I didn't have to tell him how tired I was of trying so hard to be positive when my insides were shredded. I didn't have to say that this relocation to Halifax felt like moving one step closer to his death. I didn't have to tell him how angry I was. How scared I was. How sad I was.

He knew.

Relief rushed through me, and I felt the tension under my skin ease. Dad stood and the moment retreated. He walked back toward the door. On his way by my desk he picked up my dog-eared copy of *The Grapes of Wrath*, gazed at the cover, and then set it back down. He gave my shoulder a gentle squeeze and said, "You can do this, Mel. Just get it done the best that you can."

I nodded, but I didn't speak. If I did, I'd cry.

The warm pressure of his hand against my shoulder was reassuring. After a minute, he turned to leave. I watched him go. His steps were slow and deliberate. His shoulders were bent. I picked up the book and thought of Pa Joad. The events that played out on his family's journey left his character damaged. Paralyzed. Diminished.

I propped my elbow on the desk and rested my chin in my hand. I stared again at the lined page of my notebook. After a few heavy minutes, I picked up my pen and began writing. *Pa Joad wasn't always a weakened man ...*

UNSPEAKABLE

There is no grief like the grief that does not speak.

HENRY WADSWORTH LONGFELLOW,
Hyperion

Anyway

2013

NEW ENGLAND FALL whizzed by as our Traiblazer traveled south on Interstate 93. The trees were at their peak. A festival of colors spattered the highway's rim: flaming red maples, pale yellow poplars and birches, searing orange oaks. It mingled with the signature evergreens of Northern New Hampshire. Chris, Will, Lily, and I had spent the earlier part of the day hiking up Mount Sunapee. We'd traipsed over the wet, fallen leaves and golden pine needles that carpeted the trail. Sunlight streamed through gaps in the towering canopy overhead and warmed us despite the crisp air. Our yellow Lab, Wally—the self-designated guide to the summit—ran ahead and then circled back to where we tramped over rocks and roots. The panoramic view at the top showcased the ranges of Mount Monadnock, Ragged Mountain, and Mount Kearsarge, all dressed in autumn's garments, the backdrop for our picnic lunch before we'd retraced our trek to the parking lot at the mountain's base.

Now, on the route home, the kids listened to their iPods and Wally slept, his head nestled in Lily's lap. I took advantage of the peaceful moment to call my brother Mark. I rested my elbow on the passenger door, leaned my iPhone against my ear and talked with him about the latest goings on in his world: kid activities, their house construction, work, a recent hike he'd taken with my niece Rose up Maine's Mount Katahdin. They had plans to visit Ellen's extended family for the rest of their long weekend. The US's Columbus Day is Canada's Thanksgiving.

They were headed to the annual "Duck Dinner" in Ellen's hometown of Miramichi, New Brunswick. Mark said, "I like the family gathering, but I'm always less enthused about the actual duck."

"Have you chatted with anyone else lately?" I asked.

"I talked to Mom a couple of times this week." Mark yawned his words. I could picture him on the other end of the phone, reclined on his family room couch, elbow bent behind his head, his socked feet stretching past the couch's arm, his ankles crossed. His favorite way to enjoy a quiet Saturday afternoon. A habit he'd inherited from Dad. One of many. "It sounds like she had fun with the baby." Mom had traveled to Dave and Ian's for a few days the week before to babysit my nephew, Ben, while they'd spent four days in the Bahamas. It was their first kid-free trip since becoming parents in February.

"She did," I said, "but I think she got a bit lonely after a couple of days." I shifted in my seat, an emerging ache in my right hip making it hard to get comfortable. I would feel this hike tomorrow.

"I got that impression too," Mark said. "It actually sounded like she was excited to be heading home."

There was irony in his words, and we both let them sit for a minute. The highway meandered along the banks of the Merrimack River through the city of Manchester. The trees gave way to old, red-bricked mill buildings converted into office space and upscale condos. Their over-sized windows looked out across the water.

We'd seen Mom a couple of months earlier on our yearly family vacation to Prince Edward Island. John, her husband of seven years, had chosen to stay home since he was still recovering from recent hip surgery. None of us, including Mom, had pined for his company. Since he'd joined our family, my siblings and I had struggled to warm to him. His subdued, withdrawn, and often awkward demeanor was a stark contrast to our father's charisma. Throughout the week, Mom had engaged us all in repetitive conversations about what amounted to the unhappy state of this second marriage.

"I'm ready to leave," she declared one evening as the adults lingered around the weathered picnic table after dinner, sipped glasses of wine, and listened to the echoes of the kids' voices as they played a complicated game of tag in the gathering darkness. Citronella candles in metal tins lit the faces of my brothers and their spouses around the table. The lemony scent wafted into the night, blending with briny air drifting from the ocean. I glanced at Mark and caught the end of his eye roll. I clamped down on my lips and felt my muscles stiffening. This was not a new revelation. In the last couple of years, Mom had been vocal about her discontent with John, a man she'd met, dated, and married in a total of nine months. The monotony of their life's routine of going to the gym and doing crossword puzzles was proving to be unfulfilling. We listened and offered tentative counsel, but it had become clear that Mom's words did not always mirror the reality of her day-to-day existence. She'd backpedal from these conversations with statements like, "It's not really so bad," or, "We actually do get along quite well most of the time." Nothing ever changed, and as much as we wanted to support her, the flip-flopping made it a hard conversation to navigate.

"Why don't you leave, then?" David asked in bold response to her declaration that night. He poured himself another half glass of wine and swiped a cookie off the dessert plate. He voiced the question I'd been repeating for years. Dave was gentle with his words, but I knew he shared my frustration. I loved my mother, so I wanted her to be happy. But she was the only person who could adapt her situation. Hearing the same complaints over and over again about John's indifference and sullen behavior, without a sign that anything was going to give, made me crazy. In those moments, my longing for Dad felt bottomless. He'd been the balance to any of my mother's unsteadiness. Without him, she'd struggled, and she'd rushed to find grounding in other relationships. Before John, she'd had a series of whirlwind romances that she ended as quickly as she'd started them, feeling foolish and humiliated in their wakes. I fretted that her decision to go through with this second marriage was in response to our unfiltered criticism of her past impulsivity and a refusal to admit to another failed courtship.

"I need to wait for the right time," Mom said to David. She ran her thumb along the stem of her wine glass. Her face was drawn, and indecision traced her features. "I can't just up and leave at a moment's notice."

Why not? I wanted to ask. I wanted to shake her into action and tell her to get on with things if that's what she wanted. Urge her to relieve us of the endless strain of what to feel about John and his place in our family. Was he in or was he out? I didn't want to keep living in limbo with her. I didn't want this conversation to be the same one we'd be having in a year, or in ten years. I'd voiced different versions of these thoughts in the last few years and then felt guilty for disrupting the pretense. In the flickering candlelight, I finished my wine, let my brothers offer Mom words of comfort and advice, and said nothing.

Now, a few months later, Mom had fallen back into the status quo of her life with John and, according to her, everything was "going fine." When we conversed on the phone, she presented a cheerful front. There'd been no more talk of leaving. No more talk of unhappiness. I wanted to believe that things were fine and that she was okay. But I didn't trust her words, and a lingering worry crept in whenever I thought about her pretending to like a life I knew she hated.

Chris slowed the truck and steered into the E-Z Pass lane at the Manchester tollbooths. A car ahead sported a rack with two bikes and was topped with two plastic kayaks. Traffic was heavier the farther south we got. He glanced in my direction, sensing the track of the conversation from the words on my side. He reached for my hand and gave it a squeeze.

"Apparently things are back to 'normal' on the home front," I said to Mark. I over-enunciated the word "normal" to imply that I suspected it was anything but. I wanted him to commiserate and help me shoulder some of this worry.

"You know, I think I've made my peace with it," he said. "As long as I don't have to hear about it, I'm fine," he added with a chuckle.

I'm glad you're fine, I thought. I'm glad you have peace. But what about me? I needed to talk about it. Talking was the only way I could make sense of things.

"Anyway," Mark said.

One simple word, but in my family, its use was like the checkered flag waved on a NASCAR speedway to signal the finish. When the other drivers saw it, they knew to slow down and return to their garages. The race was over.

There would be no more talking about my worry over Mom.

A familiar resignation swept through me. I pressed on my internal brakes. I swallowed my persistent fears and the sentences that had been forming to express them. I put on my own cheerful front. "Well, I hope you guys have fun in Mirimachi," I said to Mark. "Good luck trying to stomach the duck!"

"Thanks." He laughed and said, "Have a good rest of your weekend. Say hi to Chris and the kids. Love you."

"Love you too," I said and hit the red end button on my phone's touch screen. I took a deep breath and turned again in my seat to face Chris.

He raised his brows and a sympathetic smile played on his lips. "So?" he said. Chris knew how my family was and the rules of survival we'd long ago instituted. He knew that talking freely about what mattered— our troubles, our confusions, our shared pain—was not something we did often. He'd witnessed many conversations like the one with Mark where the instant things pushed beyond polite boundaries and started to get uncomfortable, the family code dictated backing off. He understood that years of hurt were buried within what had never been spoken.

Deep within the hard silences.

He also knew how much I wished that things could somehow be different.

"There's nothing to say," I responded. I stared at the colorful foliage painting the trees we passed and tried to recapture the sense of calm I'd felt earlier as we'd hiked up the quiet mountain trail. Chris squeezed my hand again.

"Anyway," I said.

What We Didn't Say

DR. B DREW the shade on his window to keep the sharp afternoon sun out of my eyes, but slivers of light sneaked through the slats and criss-crossed the space between us. Dust particles danced across their paths.

"You know what's weird?" I asked him, setting my empty Dunkin' Donuts teacup on the floor and clasping my hands together in my lap.

"What's weird?" he said.

"So much of the stuff we talk about in here is stuff I wish I could talk to my dad about." I paused, trying to shape the thought in my head into the right language on my tongue. "The weird part is that I wouldn't be talking about any of this if he was alive; I wouldn't have to." I couldn't help smiling when I added, "Because of the him being alive part and all."

Dr. B smiled too. His eyes crinkled at the corners and dimples dented his cheeks. "I get it," he said. "It makes sense that you'd want to connect with him about these painful emotions." His face grew serious again. "That's one of the biggest tragedies in your whole story for me."

"What part?"

"That you didn't feel like you could talk about the pain of your experience when your dad was alive. With either your dad or your mom."

We'd covered this territory before. More than once. It was a hard reality for me to face: the residual damage inflicted by my family's culture of silence during the ten years my dad was sick. In the nineteen years after that. Dr. B wanted me to admit that I was angry about it. Angry at my dad. He hadn't come right out and said so, but I knew that was where we were headed. There had been more than a few "What

131

did that feel like for you?"s and "How do you feel about that now?"s in our recent sessions. These standards from the therapy playbook used to make me want to run straight out his door because I was not prepared to talk about how I'd felt then or how I felt now. I'd gotten used to these questions, though, and I usually answered honestly.

Except when it came to admitting I was angry at Dad.

I didn't feel ready to do that. And I wasn't convinced that I had a right to be angry.

Among my earliest memories of my father is: Him coming through the front door of our house in Moncton, New Brunswick. It's dark outside and a cold rain patters against the windows. He's missed dinner because of an emergency that kept him late at the hospital, and a plate with a heaping portion of the chicken casserole topped with Cornflakes that Mom served the boys and me for dinner is warming in the oven under a layer of tinfoil. From where I'm perched playing with my Barbies on the hallway's carpeted floor at the top of the stairs, I see him step into the tiled entryway and brush the damp off of his navy trench coat. The bend of his shoulders and the creases in his fore-head betray his exhaustion. He carries his boxy briefcase in his left hand. Inside the case, there are cream-colored file folders with papers about his patients—"charts" he calls them when I ask what he's doing on the days he sits at his desk and, in a low voice using words I don't understand, talks into the small black handheld recorder holding tiny cassette tapes. For a moment after he walks in, Dad stands without moving, his gaze aimed forward. I have a feeling that he's not looking at anything. He pulls in a mouthful of air and blows it out again in a slow sigh.

"Hi Daddy," I say, peeking my face through the staircase's metal railing.

His eyes turn upward and a smile lights his face, erasing the tired lines. "Hi, Melanie Joybells," he says and releases his grip on the brief-case, pushing it into the corner by the door. I abandon my Barbies in a jumbled heap and dash down the stairs into his outstretched arms, feeling the wet from the rain on my cheeks. "How was your day?" he asks, kicking off his dress shoes and unbuttoning his overcoat. I launch into an account of how Madame Arsenault, my first-grade teacher, read us a story that day totally in French, and I'd understood almost every word. "It was about this brother and sister named Rémi and Aline, and they were going to their first birthday party!" I tell him as we walk toward the kitchen, my arm still stretched around his waist.

I often replay this memory and that pause in the scene when my father stood still, looking nowhere, before setting down his briefcase. What I understand now is that a shift was taking place: a moment of transition. On the other side of our front door, my father was Dr. Messenger. On this side of the door, though, he was Dad. To be Dad, he had to put down the events of his day. Put down his briefcase full of charts detailing prognoses and treatment plans and surgical outcomes and leave it, and the unrelenting stress that accompanied that work, in the entryway. He couldn't carry its weight with him into the world of our family.

My father knew how to compartmentalize his emotions, set them aside to focus on what was in front of him. I don't know if his brilliant, scientific mind was wired that way or whether he learned the skill in medical school when he was taught the art of "professional detachment" to help him cope with the distressing waves of fear, self-doubt, grief, and pain that are part of dealing with life-and-death situations every day. I don't know if the ability was learned long before then from his childhood living in the shadow of the Baptist tradition, in which Biblical directives to "fear not," to be "slow to anger," and to "not let your hearts be troubled" might have mistakenly told him displays of emotion were sinful.

What I do know is that my father's practice of coping with hard emotions became the gold standard for our family. A standard that remains intact today, twenty-five years after his death. Don't dwell. Don't look back. Let it go. And keep moving forward.

I've spent my entire life trying and failing to meet this standard. Unlike my father (and maybe my mother and my brothers) I'm not wired to put the hard things down. To let them go. I gather them all, clutching them to my chest. How was it fair for me to be angry with Dad because of my own inability to conform?

I decided to risk taking a step closer, though. "Did I ever tell you that when my parents were writing their book in those last two years before Dad died, he asked each of us kids to write down our thoughts about what it had been like for us to deal with his illness?" I asked Dr. B and stared at my hands, running my index finger along the jagged edge of a hangnail on my thumb.

Dr. B tilted his head. "I'm not sure you ever did," he said.

I told him about the night when I was twenty-one, how in the middle of dinner my father rested his fork on his plate, leaned back in his chair, and said to David and me, "I'd like you guys to write down a few thoughts about how you've felt about me being sick that I could include in the book. I'm asking Michael and Mark to do it too." He picked up his fork again and resumed eating.

I stopped chewing my food. Stunned, I looked from my father's face to my mother's, but their expressions held no hints that they viewed this request as anything out of the ordinary. I tried not to choke as I swallowed the mashed potatoes that were becoming slimy in my mouth. "Okay," I managed to respond, fighting to keep the tremor I felt throughout my body from finding its way into my voice.

Later that night, I sat at my desk, a ballpoint pen gripped in my hand, and stared at an empty, lined piece of paper. What the hell was I supposed to say? For the first time in nine years, Dad had asked me what living with the secret of his HIV had been like. Except he hadn't actually asked me to tell him in a way that would allow us to talk about it; he'd told me to write it down for him to read. I couldn't stop imagining him sitting alone at his own desk, the burden of my words and whatever words my brothers wrote, too heavy in his hands. What would that do to him? I wondered, and, for days, the ache in the question kept me from writing anything.

"Eventually," I said to Dr. B, "I wrote a few things down because I knew if I didn't write something, he'd have to ask me again."

"What did you write?" he asked.

"Not the truth," I said. My jaw tightened.

His raised brows questioned my statement.

"I don't mean I lied," I rushed to say. I was forever wondering what Dr. B was thinking, and despite his constant reassurance that I was allowed to say anything to him, I had this fear that he might think badly of me. "I wrote about true experiences. True moments. But I chose my words carefully." I told him I'd written some brief snapshots that touched on incidents when my understanding of AIDS broadened or my recognition of how it impacted some of our family interactions was clear. I wrote about my parents' suffering and their courage as they faced the unknowns of the disease together. "I just didn't write how it really felt to be living with the secret. The uncertainty. How painful it really was. How lonely I felt. How confused and frightened."

"Why not?"

I looked at him and said, "We'd never talked about those things. And here he was asking us to write it down and give it to him. How could I do that? Throw all those feelings at him on a scrap of paper? It must have been devastating for him to read the things we wrote."

"He didn't talk about it after you gave him what you'd written?" Dr. B asked.

"No."

A bitter taste filled my mouth as I recounted how I'd slipped into the basement den that housed Dad's oak computer desk and deposited next to his keyboard the five handwritten pages that had taken me over four hours to finish. In the weeks that followed, he hadn't said a word about them, and I hadn't asked. I had no idea what he'd done with the pages until the first time I read a printed manuscript of the book a few months later and came to the chapter titled, "Reflections—Dad Has AIDS." There, positioned among excerpts written by my brothers, were neatly typed paragraphs that quoted my words from those hand-written pages.

I had been feeling at odds with Dad for a number of things ... One day, after a particularly heated confrontation, I remember Mom turning to me and saying, "Don't you realize that he just wants to be sure you are all okay because he knows he may not be around to see the final product?" ... Finally, I understood what had been happening around me for so long. And for the first time, I understood my parents' pain—because I felt it, too.

There were individuals on campus who somehow had heard through the grapevine about my dad ... I felt violated, in a sense, because these were people with whom I was barely acquainted but who somehow knew my most intimate secret.

In a situation that could have torn them apart, Mom and Dad's love for each other has gotten stronger. I watch them take advantage of every moment they have together.

There are times when I see Mom's grief and feel physically sick at the loss she has yet to face. These are emotions for which my Christian faith has largely been unable to provide solace.

In their personal accounts, my brothers detailed moments and experiences when they had to cope with the grief and insecurity of Dad's illness. Things that we'd never talked about before. Instinct told me that we'd never talk about them after, either.

I still remember the evening that we sat down in the family room and Dad told us about the infected blood transfusion ... A sense of numbness descended over us all; even eight years later that feeling has never really disappeared.

It is tempting, and true, to say that we have been blessed to have Dad alive and reasonably healthy for nine full years. But they have been years lived day to day; sometimes the specter of disaster is more difficult to deal with than if it were confirmed reality.

I try not to dwell on Dad being sick all of the time. There are times when I won't think of it at all—I'll just sort of let it slide into the shadows and go on with my life. Other times, it's on my mind a lot ...

My father had prefaced the chapter with: *The illness of a family member creates suffering for all other family members. The extent of that suffering for each of our children is difficult to gauge; it's not a subject we talk about often.*

"It wasn't a subject we talked about *ever*," I told Dr. B. I wrapped my arms around my body, trying to restrain the rush of feeling spreading through me.

Dr. B knew my therapy mannerisms. Knew when to adjust our course enough to give me a reprieve from emotions that felt too big. He leaned back, quiet for a minute, clasping and unclasping the silver watch on his wrist before he launched into an unexpected personal story. "In the days after my mother died, my brother and sister and I decided to go through some of her things while we were all still together in Maine—organizing rooms, making plans for eventually clearing out the house. I opened a drawer in one of her bureaus and found stacks of her journals, full of stories and important events from her life." He paused, and a suggestion of grief crossed his features. "I picked up one of the journals on top and read the date. 2010. The year after my father died. I opened to the first page. She'd titled it: *The Year of My Loneliness.*" Dr. B's voice took on a tenor of sadness as he described how the journal chronicled his mother's intense anguish in the wake of losing her husband of over fifty years.

His eyes glistened with tears. "It broke my heart. I had no idea how much she was suffering."

Tears brimmed in my eyes too. The portrait of this solitary woman letting her burden of sorrow seep from her pen to the page was both tender and painful.

"I imagine you wish you could have helped her," I said softly.

"I do," he said. "But more than that, I wish she'd shared her sadness with us so we could have shared ours." He was giving me that pointed look of his. "Then," he said, his voice soft too, "we could have all walked through the pain together."

The Official Story
1994

"I THOUGHT YOU might want to read this," Dad said, holding out a thick sheaf of printed computer paper fastened together by a large, black binder clip. "It's done."

He stood on the carpeted landing midway down the staircase that led to the finished basement and my bedroom. He was dressed in a pair of baggy sweats and a fuzzy, fleece pullover. His feet were bare. I'd been on my way to my room for the night, planning to change into my own sweats and catch up on some schoolwork for my graduate classes. He'd startled me when he appeared in the doorway just as I was about to duck around the corner through my bedroom door. I thought he'd gone to bed.

I turned and started back up the stairs as he made his way down, and we met in the middle. Nothing on his face betrayed any emotion, and his tone was matter-of-fact, but I felt the heightened intensity of his look as I reached for the pages and took them in my hands. They felt heavy.

"The Book?" I asked, my voice a little breathless.

"The Book," he said before turning and heading back the way he'd come. His gait was slow as he climbed the steps.

I stood there after he disappeared through the doorway and stared at the stack of paper. Curiosity and hesitation overlapped and for a minute I wasn't sure what to do. That these pages existed was a miracle. Three months earlier, standing in the same spot, I'd been convinced they never would.

The cursor blinked on the screen, the rhythmic vertical line the only contrast to the expanse of grayish blankness. A sick feeling grew in my gut.

The Book was gone.

David sat in the leather desk chair in my parents' finished basement and continued opening documents and files, sliding the mouse along the pad, typing on the keyboard. He was pretending to search. Delaying the inevitable. From where I stood behind him, I read the anxiety in his rigid shoulders and clenched jaw. It leached into the air and squeezed.

Dad stood beside Dave, and his hand rested on the dark wood of the desk. Hope still lit his face—hope that David, with his superior computer knowledge, could recover the lost document.

He couldn't.

I knew it. Dave knew it. And in another minute, Dad would know it too.

The project began a few months earlier, in October 1993, when Dad went on a solo camping trip to Kejumkujik National Park, two hours from our home in Halifax. He used this retreat to start writing about having AIDS, a personal, therapeutic attempt to organize and understand the mess of what had happened to him. When he returned, he continued to write to fill the empty days of his new and unwelcome retirement that arrived earlier that year when debilitating fatigue, constant headaches, and more frequent bouts with opportunistic infections forced him to stop his work with the Canadian Medical Protective Association.

As his narrative took shape, he read passages to my mother, and she added thoughts of her own. An idea bloomed between them: Maybe they had something to say. Maybe their experience living with HIV and AIDS could help someone else. Maybe their unique story could dispel some of the myths that swirled in the AIDS climate of the early 1990s and add a different voice to the mix. Maybe their story mattered enough to break a nine-year silence and spill their secret. Our secret.

I was living at home for the year before Chris and I got married, completing a graduate program in education at Dalhousie University, a ten-minute drive from the house. Often, I'd arrive home from school in the early afternoon and stand in the empty kitchen, listening to the hum of Dad's voice drifting up through the floorboards from the basement. He dictated and Mom typed, interjecting when she had added pieces to include.

I didn't interrupt. My parents made no great pronouncement of what they were doing to my brothers and me, but they weren't hiding it either. We tread carefully around the concept of The Book. Writing this story was a risk for Dad. A risk I'd never dreamed he'd take. I didn't push and only asked questions when Dad talked about it himself. The last thing I wanted to do was frighten him back into the shadows. Even though I shared the same desktop computer to write papers for school, I didn't open the file labeled *Book* to sneak a look at what they were writing. To me, the endeavor felt precarious, like a fragile cord being woven together, thin thread by thin thread, to create a lifeline that could finally pull us out of our isolation.

So, when I'd walked through the garage door into the house earlier that afternoon and Dad stood in the kitchen greeting my arrival with the words: "Mel, I need your help with something on the computer. I can't find my document," my insides constricted.

I followed Dad down the stairs to the finished basement. The wood stove was burning, toasting the room. Abby, our Golden Retriever, reclined against the stone hearth. She lifted her head from where it rested on a pillow to acknowledge our arrival and gave us three thumps of her tail before closing her eyes once more. Mom was away for a few days visiting my aunt and my grandmother in Ontario, so while David and I were at school, it was just Dad, the dog, and The Book.

"I was making some changes to some of the pages Mom typed earlier this week," Dad said, standing to the side so I could sit down in front of the computer. I shook the mouse attached to the boxy monitor and began scrolling through the files in the WordPerfect folder. "I took a break for lunch, and when I went back to open it, something happened." He didn't define what the "something" was. Dad's computer skills were not among his best assets.

I'd clicked on the document and prayed silently as the file loaded. *Please be there. Please be there.* As with so many others, my prayer went unanswered. A blank page opened on the screen. I scrolled to the bottom to find nothing but more blankness.

"Did you maybe save it under a different name?" I asked, opening other documents—Dave's homework assignments, my lesson plans for student teaching. I already knew the answer. As I searched, I replayed what I guessed had happened. Dad had opened the file, worked on it, and went to close the document but hit a mistaken key. An unusual message opened asking if he wanted to proceed with the action. Assuming he was saving his document, he clicked *yes.* He erased the whole thing and left behind an empty file.

My eyes traced the vertical pattern of the wood paneling on the walls. I couldn't bring myself to turn around and look into Dad's expectant face. I didn't know what to do. "I think you might have los ..." I began, but my admission was cut short by the sound of a slamming door, footsteps overhead, and a bellowed "Hello?" from the top of the stairs. David was home from school.

"Down here, Dave," Dad shouted. "We need you!" His voice remained cheerful. He didn't know what he'd done yet. He trusted David to swoop in and figure things out. But after scrolling and typing and searching for close to an hour, David had not figured things out.

The Book was gone.

Dave swiveled the desk chair toward me, and our eyes met. The question wedged between us. Who was going to tell him?

"Dad," Dave said, his voice strained. He pushed back the chair. "It looks like you accidentally erased the file."

It was a few seconds before Dad absorbed the words.

"I. Did. Not." Dad's face contorted. His body stiffened. Rage soaked into each syllable. "You must have done something, David! You spend too much time screwing around on this computer! You did something."

The accusation landed hard on David's shoulders. He slouched into the seat, his pained eyes downcast. He tried to protest, tried to explain what must have happened, but Dad moved away from us both. As quickly as it flared, his anger dissipated. Weariness settled in its place. "Well, that's it then," he said. The harsh finality of the statement hit like a slap.

Dad didn't look at David or me. His eyes had clouded into an expression I'd never seen before, and he'd retreated somewhere unreachable inside his head. He walked out of the room, Abby at his feet, and climbed the stairs, his fatigue more pronounced with every step.

For a few agonizing weeks, Dad refused to talk about The Book, and a veil of grim defeat settled over the household. The hope I'd been feeling flamed out. I assumed the potential of inviting others into our story was gone.

Then, one day, I returned from school and found Mom and Dad sitting once again together in front of the computer. Dad grasped a bundle of papers in his hands. He read slowly, "April 14, 1985 was a beautiful Sunday afternoon, cold with snow still on the ground ..." and Mom typed. They both turned to look at me when I walked into the room. "You're not going to believe this," Dad said and held up the papers in triumph. "Mom was cleaning this morning and found this folder behind the computer monitor!"

"It's all of Dad's handwritten journal pages from when he first started," Mom chimed in, her smile broad. "We both thought he threw them away after we transferred it all to the computer."

"Turns out it's about sixty percent of what we had," Dad explained, his face flushed and animated. I felt the tremor as a small internal spark reignited.

— ❦ —

Three months later, I leaned back on my bed in my basement room and let my aching shoulders sink into the pile of mismatched throw pillows. I clutched The Book to my chest and tried to sort out the thoughts unspooling in my brain. In the dim light cast by the small reading lamp clamped to the headboard, I stared at the grid of square tiles on the ceiling. Two floors above, my parents and David were sleeping, but even though it was close to 2 a.m., I was wide awake.

Moments before, I'd turned the last page of the manuscript Dad gave me earlier that evening. For six hours, I sat cross-legged on the center of my mattress, reading my parents' carefully crafted narrative of what our family had been through since Dad's infection in 1985. I read and re-read passages until the sentences smudged on the crisp, white pages. Despite having been present for it all, I felt like I was on the outside looking in on the story they told. The revelations in the book that exposed my parents' pain—the fear and desperation they'd lived with that, until now, had been hidden from my view—splintered me.

More than once, my father had considered suicide as an alternative to the unknown trajectory of his disease. *I carried sufficient drugs in my medical kit that could have ended my life quickly,* he wrote. He'd battled debilitating depression and lain awake anxious in the night because he couldn't stop thinking about how he was going to die. He'd raged at God and floundered in his attempts to figure out how his Christian faith connected to the cruelty of his circumstances. *But AIDS—what possible explanation for this? It completely floored me—this disaster seemed so merciless.* He'd lost the vocation he loved and with it, he'd lost not only his identity, but also his self-confidence. *Something of myself is missing and as a result, I feel less of a person,* he wrote. Since his diagnosis, my mother had borne the crushing burden of being my father's sole confidante, and, because my father was terrified of the dangers of disclosure, she could never seek the support she needed. So, alone, she'd shouldered his suffering and her own. *Sometimes I feel like I'm up and down on the same roller coaster as he is,* she'd written.

I gripped the manuscript tighter, squeezing against my own deepening sadness. For nine years, my family had kept the secret of Dad's illness from the rest of the world, and I knew why.

But my parents had reasons for hiding so much of their personal trauma even within the walls of our home. When they learned of Dad's diagnosis, they sat down with Michael and Mark and explained what was happening. They did not tell David or me. I solved the puzzle early on, but for seven of those nine years, David, who was only eight when Dad was infected, didn't know. We were all complicit in keeping up the façade of a "normal" life for him, and I think my parents believed the less they said to the rest of us, the more normal our lives could be too.

Life was anything but normal.

Even though my parents didn't talk about their torment directly with me, I felt it. I'd never forget David's words to me when I spoke to him on the phone from my college dorm room after I learned my parents had finally revealed the secret to him. "So much of my life makes sense to me now."

Now, with the contents of the book transcribed to my brain, I, too, could name the anguish of those nine years.

But the burn of something deeper than my parents' revelations of their trauma was rising in me. Why did it matter that I hadn't known the intimate details of their suffering as it happened? What could I have done for them?

I wanted this question to propel me from this troubled landing after finishing the manuscript to a place of resolution. A place where I could excuse all they'd never said.

Instead, another question loomed larger than the first. What could they have done *for me*?

I closed my eyes, and a stampede of painful memories pounded across my eyelids. I pictured so many other nights like the one before our move to Ottawa when I could not fall asleep because I couldn't stop thinking about how Dad would die. I remembered times when friends were spilling secrets, and all I wanted to talk about was the one I'd been forbidden to tell. I thought of the relief I felt the night in the yellow Camaro when I broke the rules and told Gene about Dad. I replayed the endless prayers that felt ignored by the God I'd always trusted.

I sat up again and set the stack of pages down in front of me on the white eyelet comforter. I rubbed my eyes and started from the beginning, slowly turning one page after another, skimming the lines for my name. Apart from minor mentions of where I was at points in time, I didn't find anything until almost fifty pages into the story. In a chapter that described the first year after my father's diagnosis when we'd moved a thousand miles across the country to Ontario and away from the only home I'd ever known in New Brunswick, Dad wrote:

Melanie, within three months of arriving in town, had won the Junior Public Speaking award for the Ottawa/Carleton region. Every time we turned on our local public television channel, there was Melanie on the umpteenth rerun of the competition with her speech entitled "TV Commercials"! It gave her recognition that she needed in her new situation, and oblivious to our dreary accommodations, she remained her sunny self. We have always felt that Melanie has a special gift of cheerfulness that the family has drawn upon regularly as a source of strength.

I pressed my finger to the page and used my nail to draw a dim line underneath certain words as I reread the paragraph.

Oblivious to our dreary accommodations ...

Remained her sunny self ...

Gift of cheerfulness ...

Source of strength ...

A hollow formed in my chest as the air left my lungs in an extended, audible sigh. I lifted my eyes to the surrounding dark and pictured that sunny, thirteen-year-old girl.

She stood in the living room of a small, rented bungalow, crowded with faded furniture that smelled like old people, listening to her beloved father repeat the opening of her speech about television commercials he'd been feverishly rewriting since she'd shown him the draft assignment for her grade eight Language Arts class.

"Like this, Mel," he said from his seat on the couch. Enthusiasm she hadn't heard from him in months energized his voice. "Have you ever heard the phrase, 'Where's the beef?' Does the name 'Herb' ring a bell? Have *you* driven a Ford lately?" He sat back against the cushions and waited.

She smoothed her hands down the front of her plaid, woolen skirt, took a deep breath, and repeated the lines, imitating the rise and fall of his tone and putting emphasis on the same words he had.

Her father leaned forward and propped his hands on his knees. His eyes were alive behind his square, plastic rimmed glasses, and his face creased into a deep smile, something else she hadn't seen much of lately. "Yes! Yes!" he said. "You've got it!"

She smiled, too, clinging to his pleasure as though it were a life raft. She felt some of the heaviness leak from the surrounding air.

"Ready to try the next part?" her father asked.

She resolved to do anything to keep that smile on his face a while longer.

"Absolutely," she said and waited for him to script her next words.

The girl's image faded, and I refocused my attention on scanning the pages. As it turned out, this was the one and only place where my parents had written directly about me. How, when I remembered so much more about this girl, was this singular portrait of her all my parents had seen? A small voice at the back of my consciousness answered: *This was all they'd wanted to see.*

By contrast, in writing about my older brothers' experiences, they acknowledged elements of their trauma:

[Friends from our church] gave Michael the support he needed badly just weeks after learning of my test results, and away from home for the first time ... We were very proud of Michael—he had weathered a lonely time.

Mark had a tough time in his cold basement room ... Mark missed his brother and his old friends. He tried not to add his problems to our worries, but we knew.

I swept my arm across the stack of pages on my bed and pushed it to the floor. Save for a few of the top sheets that fluttered across the carpet, the manuscript settled with a thud. I stared into the blank spot where The Book had been. Something more belonged in that white space, but I didn't yet know what.

My parents would publish this "official" version of the story in less than a year, only six months before Dad's death. For two weeks, it would appear on the Toronto *Globe and Mail*'s bestseller list. As we'd hoped, it would prompt an unexpected and compassionate response of support for my parents from family, friends, colleagues, and strangers around the country—a response that I'd mostly miss out on because, by then, I'd be married and moved away, my own unwritten version of the story still trapped beneath thick layers of denial and secrecy.

I climbed under the comforter, pulling it to my chin. I reached for the off switch on the reading lamp, and the night swallowed me. I stared again toward the ceiling, straining my eyes to see into the darkness until they stung with tears.

"I wish you'd told me before now," I whispered. "Because maybe then, I could have told you too."

How to Walk Together
2014

LILY IS AFRAID of big trucks on the highway. Our neighbor once told her the gruesome details of an accident involving an eighteen-wheeler and the SUV belonging to a friend of her mother's, which had careened underneath the truck, peeling away the car's roof and killing the passengers. The story planted itself in Lily's imagination. In vivid, Technicolor detail, Lily's brain can recreate scenes she's never witnessed and make them as real to her as her own lived experiences. She's like me that way.

I was not surprised to hear her voice this fear more than once on a weekend trip to Burlington, Vermont. Interstate 89 travels north from New Hampshire through Vermont to the Canadian border and serves as a transport route for many commercial vehicles carrying freight between Boston and Montreal. Many tractor trailers shared the road with us. Every time we saw one, Lily closed her eyes and told me to hurry up and drive past "because," she reminded me with a dramatic sigh, "I really hate big trucks!"

Lily and her best friend, Kate, were nestled in the backseat of our Traverse, their blonde heads resting against their pillows, their bodies cuddled underneath a fleece blanket. They were watching the sing-along version of *High School Musical* on the pop-down movie screen and up until a few minutes ago their voices had belted out the familiar songs. Now they watched quietly, betraying their exhaustion. We were headed home after two intense days of soccer. Earlier, Lily and

Kate's U-13 travel team missed winning the championship game of the annual Nordic Cup Tournament by one goal. Their team played hard in all five of their games—better than they'd played all season— so no one wallowed in disappointment. The girls had a blast spending the weekend together, and the bonding with their team off the field—swimming in the hotel pool and going out to eat—had been as much fun for them as the soccer games.

I took the girls by myself to the tournament. Chris stayed home with Will, and Kate's parents were traveling for a family function. I was starting to feel my own exhaustion setting in, an inevitable one that came after spending sixty hours straight with two tween girls. I shifted my position in the seat, stretched my back and neck, and gazed lazily at the towering evergreens whizzing past. The weather had been sunny and warm most of the weekend, but now, a gray, cloud-filled sky reached across the surrounding peaks of the Green Mountains. Rain was in the forecast.

I startled to a deafening boom. Large pieces of rubber tire tread flew out from beneath the semi-truck we were following and missed our car by inches. The truck fishtailed from one side of the double-lane highway to the other, crossing into the gravel breakdown lane, and appeared dangerously close to overturning. I gripped the steering wheel, concentrated on staying in our lane and braked to keep us at a safe distance. The truck stopped swerving, began to slow, and moved to the right lane, its yellow hazard lights flashing. I switched lanes and coasted by, my knuckles still white on the wheel, my heartbeat pounding in my ears. Once we were past, I exhaled and released my shoulders.

"Everybody okay?" I asked, glancing at the girls in the rearview mirror.

They removed their headphones and sat stiff in their seats. Kate nodded, but Lily's face was a white marble, her hazel eyes spheres of panic. "Mama," she said, her voice small and trembling.

Lily's fear was palpable to me, a pressure that filled the car and pushed relentlessly against my body. I longed to push back with familiar platitudes: *There's nothing to worry about. Everything's fine. It's not that big a deal. Stop thinking about it. Focus on something else. Don't be afraid.* I wanted to throw these last words over her like a veil. To shield her from all the scary things. To just keep driving.

But the scary thing had happened. Saying those words wouldn't extract the images of the swerving truck or the flying tire tread from Lily's mind. Telling her not to be afraid wasn't going to change the fact that she already was.

I believe my parents imagined that keeping silent about their terror about my father's illness and looming death was a protective veil they were throwing over me. But I also recognize that keeping silent about my terror was a veil they were throwing over themselves. In this moment when Lily's fear was so big, and all I wanted to do was sidestep it, I understood that impulse.

Instead, I said, "Hold on," and signaled toward the upcoming exit ramp. As soon as we were off the highway, I pulled into a gravel lot and stopped the car. I undid my seatbelt and turned to the backseat. I reached for Lily's hand and felt her blood pulsing through her fingers. I gave them a squeeze. "I'm here," I said. And then, "It's okay, you guys. Let's just breathe for a second." I inhaled a full breath and then slowly let it out. They followed my lead, and I watched the slack return to their bodies.

"What *was* that, Miss Melanie?" Kate asked, her voice a little shaky too.

"The truck's tire blew," I said. "The good news is that those kinds of trucks have a lot of tires, so losing one isn't necessarily a disaster."

"It was crazy loud," Kate said. "I thought it was a gunshot!"

"That was like my worst nightmare come true," Lily exclaimed, the residual adrenaline now making her breathless and animated. "You guys know how much I *hate* trucks, and that's exactly why!"

"We *do* know," I said. "But you are okay. We are okay. The truck driver is okay. And, luckily, there weren't any other cars nearby, so I could slow down and get out of the way. We really are okay. But," I gave Lily's hand another squeeze. "That was totally scary."

"Right?" Lily's cheeks pinked up. I left my hand in hers until she was ready to let it go. Soon, she settled back into her seat, nudging a bit closer to Kate. "Can we get something to eat?"

"Sure," I said and clicked my seatbelt into the buckle. "Let's get back on the highway and look for the next exit with fast food. I think we all need some French fries."

DYING LIGHT

Do not go gentle into that good night.
Rage, rage against the dying of the light.

DYLAN THOMAS,
"Do Not Go Gentle Into That Good Night"

Everything Feels Tenuous
2013

"I KEEP HAVING a version of this dream about you," I said to Dr. B one day, and heat flooded my face as soon as the statement left my lips. Flustered, I stumbled to qualify, "It's nothing weird or anything. Don't get the wrong idea." I sank deeper into the couch, tucking my arms against my ribcage, trying to make myself as small as possible. Things had gotten awkward.

Dr. B grinned at my attempt to disguise my discomfort. "Why don't you just tell me about it?" he said.

I had to keep reminding myself that there was not much I could say in here that would shock him. I mean, take the guy whose appointment was before mine, the one with the eye-patch who still managed to notice and compliment the color of my clothing every time he walked by me in the waiting room. I nicknamed him The Pirate. Surely his admissions were more risqué than mine.

Then there was the middle-aged woman with the thick-lensed glasses and the ginormous bag—about the size of a beach bag—who sat across from me in those few minutes of waiting before Dr. B showed me to his office. As I imagined her situation, I'd decided the bag held props. And anyone who brought props to therapy definitely had more interesting things to say than I did.

I tamped down on my urge to interrupt myself and ask Dr. B where I ranked on the Scale of Crazy compared to the other clients he saw. The likelihood of him telling me was minimal.

"You actually don't make a real appearance in the dream," I said, instead. "It's really your absence that creates the problem." I relaxed into the telling. In each of the dreams, the opening scene was the same: I showed up at Dr. B's office for my scheduled appointment. I walked through the street-facing entrance to the building and climbed the carpeted staircase, my hand gliding along the metal railing. When I reached the landing, I paused outside the closed door and dug through my purse for my iPhone, pulling it out and pushing down the button on the side to make it silent before reaching for the knob. I pushed the door open and stepped into the waiting room.

"The first time I had the dream, I walked in and everything was missing," I said.

"How so?" Dr. B asked, curiosity bending his brows.

"It was all gone. The chairs and tables in the waiting room. The pictures on the wall. The coat rack. The water cooler. Everything. The space was completely empty."

In the dream, I'd started to panic—that exaggerated this-is-a-dream-so-it-feels-much-worse-than-maybe-it-is panic. My heart hammered a drum in my ears and my breath released in quick, strangled gasps. Swallowing my mounting dread, I pressed on down the short hallway to Dr. B's office. The door was ajar, and when I walked in, there was nothing left in that space either. Even the window blinds had been removed, the chipped holes in the drywall, the only remnants of their mountings. I stood for a long time in the middle of the room, its emptiness mirroring my own.

That same emptiness settled over me now as I described the scene.

Dr. B inclined his head to the side and his expression turned thoughtful. "You said that was how it played out the first time," he responded. "What happens in the other versions?"

"In those, the office hasn't been cleared out, but I sit in the waiting room long past our appointment time expecting you to come and get me. You don't. Eventually, someone—your office manager, I think—comes and tells me you don't work here anymore."

He didn't say anything at first, and I started to feel stupid, wishing I hadn't presented this unfiltered view into my subconscious for him to scrutinize. Like so many other moments in here, it felt risky.

"You're waiting for me to leave, aren't you?" he said, his voice quiet. There was nothing accusatory in the question. In fact, it was not really a question. More like a revelation he'd stumbled upon.

"It's not you," I said, an apology perched on my lips. "It's just that ... it's because I don't ... I want to ..." I tripped on my words. Dumb tears threatened at the backs of my eyes, and I supported my elbows on my knees, my knuckles pressed against my lips.

It had taken me countless weekly sessions sitting across from Dr. B to chisel an opening into the fortress that housed my most conflicted emotions—the ones that I was still trying to name. I also understood that my experience wasn't unique or revolutionary. Opening up in therapy was hard for everyone, I suspected. It was just that I was exceptionally practiced at keeping things to myself.

"It's like I'm on the operating table," I sputtered in desperation. "On the table, with my chest open, my ribs spread apart, my damaged heart exposed." I hesitated then, aware that I hadn't drawn this metaphor from my imagination.

"You think I might not stay with you until you're put back together," Dr. B said, nodding to the cadence of his words.

I couldn't speak. The tears were too close, so I nodded too.

"I don't have any plans to go anywhere," he said. As usual, his tone was kind and reassuring, excruciatingly so.

I knew he meant it, and I wished that him meaning it were enough to make me set aside my fears. But I was still reeling from the fourth dream. The one from two nights ago.

The one I couldn't tell him about because this one he was in.

It began exactly like the first: I arrived. The waiting room was cleared out. Panic set in. I walked down the hall. Only this time, when I pushed the door of his office open, I saw him on the floor. His body still. I knew immediately that he was dead because his eyes, the hub of all his warmth, were iced marbles, blank and staring at nothing.

"Help!" I screamed. "I need help!" I dropped to my knees and pounded my fist against his rigid chest, over and over, until my arm was numb and aching, and I couldn't lift it anymore. It didn't matter, though. There was nothing I could do.

This was what I wanted to say now: I'm not waiting for you to leave. That's not how it works for me. I'm expecting something will take you away. Something you and I will both be powerless to stop.

But how could I tell him that I'd dreamed he died? How could I tell him that the way I felt about the possibility of him leaving had gotten snarled with all the old feelings of helplessness about my dad? It was too intimate. And maybe too morbid to say out loud.

"I'll be right here for as long as it takes you to work through these things, okay?" Dr. B reiterated.

Even if it takes forever?

Mainstay
1995

"I WANT PIE," the words began at a whisper. Dad straightened in the plastic deck chair and shifted his body forward. He squeezed both hands into fists, held them in the air, gave me a mischievous wink, and then pounded them against the glass patio table in a repeating rhythm. "Bring me pie! Give me pie! I want pie!" he chanted to the beat, his voice getting louder. His laughter rang in the breaks between his words.

From where she stood inside the screen door, my mother said, "Orv, you know you can't." A note of exasperation in her voice masked her worry.

"Don't eat anything while you are gone, Dr. Messenger!" the floor nurse had commanded a few hours earlier when she'd unhooked Dad's IV drip, then covered with a wide bandage the tube that wound from the butterfly needle in his hand, and watched with resigned disapproval as he'd prepared for this temporary leave from the hospital. He'd slipped on his shoes, grabbed my arm and shuffled out of his room and into the corridor.

"Don't worry," he promised the nurse over his shoulder. "I won't." He almost sounded convincing. Turning to me, his smile planting deep grooves in his cheeks, his eyes sparking to life, he said, "Get me out of here!"

On this late June day, the air was fresh and the sun warmed my bare arms. The perfect temperature to relax on the back deck off my parents' home perched on a ravine overlooking the broad expanse of Halifax Harbor. The breath of a breeze wafted around us, but far down on the water, boats with billowing sails drifted beneath the two suspension bridges connecting Halifax Peninsula to Dartmouth. Small, colorful triangles bobbed on white-capped waves.

"C'mon, Dorsie," Dad pleaded. "Just let me scrape the plate." He'd caught sight of the remnants of last night's dessert when we'd guided him through the kitchen upon our arrival from the hospital. A tin plate covered in plastic wrap on the counter held the last sliver of home-made strawberry pie.

Dad loved pie, and fruit pies were Mom's specialty. There'd always been a tacit rule in our house that stretched back to the years when nights on call forced Dad to miss dinner: the final piece of pie was reserved for him. He'd eat it straight out of the pan every time. A late-night snack. An indulgent breakfast. One of his favorite things was to scrape up every bit of the soggy pastry swimming in the sugary juice that remained.

"What's the harm, Mom?" I asked from where I reclined in my deck chair across the table. I didn't know the answer to my question. Chris and I had only arrived two days ago from Baltimore to celebrate David's high school graduation. I hadn't been witness to the severe stomach pain that had put Dad in the hospital after a long night with Mom and Mark in the Emergency Room right before we got there. But letting him savor his favorite things felt important these days.

Dad saw he was gaining leverage. He turned in his seat toward the other faces around the table. "I want pie!" he chanted, looking from Chris to David to Ellen and finally resting his gaze on Mark, the doctor. The look in Dad's eyes said: *Help me out here, son.*

"Give him the pie, Mom," Mark said, amused resignation in his words.

When Mom turned and headed toward the kitchen, Dad leaned back in his chair with an impish look of satisfaction plastering his face.

Mom emerged a minute later, carrying the pie plate and a fork. She set them down in front of Dad with a sigh. "You're hopeless." She rested her hand on his shoulder before she sat in the empty chair beside him.

Dad cut into the flaky pastry and balanced a large hunk on the fork. His eyes lit as he moved it toward his mouth. Just before his lips circled the bite, a rogue strawberry fell and bounced down the front of his white button-down shirt and landed at his feet. A dripping trail of bright red juice that immediately seeped into the cotton fabric followed behind.

"Well," Dad said, undeterred as he popped the rest of the bite into his mouth and scooped up another. "I'm going to be needing a new shirt before I head back because that won't be easy to hide from the nurses."

Our laughter joined his and pealed across the treetops. It caught on the late afternoon breeze and floated toward the enclosed bay of the Bedford Basin below.

This was not Dad's first or last jailbreak of the week.

Much to his chagrin, he'd been diagnosed with a bowel obstruction and had been in the hospital for the previous few days. He was being monitored for any other possible infections and only allowed IV fluids. This was the first time (and only, it would turn out) that he'd been hospitalized during the nine-and-a-half years since his HIV infection, and he was doing his best to live up to the reputation that doctors make horrible patients. Case in point, his afternoon escape and pie smuggling.

Dad was the beating heart of our family. He was the planner, the leader, the go-to guy—especially when there was an important event or someone was visiting. This week with David's graduation and our arrival, there were both. Normally, he'd have our visit planned from start to finish: a dinner out at Five Fisherman, my favorite restaurant in Halifax with its all you could eat mussel bar; a drive out to Peggy's Cove to wander over the giant boulders and watch the waves crash against the rocky ledges under the lighthouse; additional celebratory activities leading up to David's graduation. To be stuck in a sterile hospital room attached to an IV pole was akin to torture for him. He was determined that our visit would not be about sitting around watching him and bemoaning the fact that he was sick.

So, he refused to be sick. He'd call the house and convince whoever picked up the phone to break him out for a few hours at a time. His doctor was a friend, so he was more lenient about these daily departures than he might have been for another patient, as long as Dad followed the rules and came back when he got tired.

Late the afternoon before, when Chris and I called to say we'd made it to Halifax, instead of having us drive to the hospital to see him, Dad told us to send Mom to come and get him and for us to meet them at the waterfront. "Tell her to bring my sneakers, so I can walk with you guys. There's a whole new area that's opened since you were here last!" he said before hanging up.

Chris and I took our own car along the Bedford Highway toward downtown Halifax while Mom went and "sprung" Dad. We drove past the container terminal where huge, international cargo ships docked and offloaded rectangular containers onto waiting freight trains that chugged in the opposite direction from where we were headed. We passed the Fairview Cemetery. Somewhere at its center, three rows of rectangular granite markers memorialized the graves of more than one hundred victims of the *Titanic*. Though most of the survivors were sailed to New York, it was Halifax-based ships that recovered many of the bodies, and those victims of the tragedy found their final resting places in three of Halifax's cemeteries. Forty-two of the stones for victims who were never identified were marked only with the date of death. I'd visited the site only once, and these unmarked graves, in particular, had filled me with sadness. What missing stories did they hold?

As Chris merged onto Barrington Street and followed the peninsula into downtown proper, an uneasy feeling rose in my stomach. "I'm nervous," I said.

"Why?" he asked, glancing in my direction. He downshifted as he maneuvered behind a line of cars.

"I'm afraid to see him sick," I said. Dad had been "sick" for almost ten years, but the physical symptoms of his illness had always been hidden. Things were changing.

"It'll be okay," Chris said with his usual calm. He said that a lot.

He turned into the parking lot off of Lower Water Street, where we were meeting Mom and Dad. Dad stood waiting for us, his body leaning against the car. I'd seen him just two months earlier when he and Mom visited us in Baltimore and took us for a weekend trip to North Carolina. I hadn't known it then, but Mom confided in me later that, during the trip, he'd started having night sweats that soaked the bed sheets. The first telltale signs that his illness was progressing. I could see he was thinner now. Hollows caved in his cheeks, and the angular lines of his neck and back seemed more pronounced. Something in the stoop of his shoulders spoke to a new weakness. I looked at Chris as he pulled into the empty parking spot beside them. He pressed his hand to my leg but said nothing.

Dad's face flooded with joy as I stepped out of the car. "Hello, Meligans!" he bellowed and folded me into a hug. Even with the new frailty in his frame, I felt the presence and security of his dad-strength as I settled into the squeeze. Despite being twenty-three, married for a year, and living far away, my axis point still hinged to that space in his arms.

"How are you doing?" I asked as casually as I could, but a note of concern crept into my voice anyway.

"I'm fine. Fine. Just an inconvenience. Bad timing. I'll be home in a couple of days," he deflected. He turned to Chris, shook his hand and patted him on the shoulder.

"If you actually follow the rules," my mother warned, holding his arm as we started toward the entrance to the boardwalk.

As a working port, the Halifax waterfront was a bustling area with shops, restaurants, and museums connected by a boarded walkway that stretched for about three kilometers along the water. Container ships traveled the waterway to and from the north end cargo terminal, a commuter ferry ran every fifteen minutes across the water to Dartmouth, and in the summer, the harbor was speckled with pleasure boats, chartered tours, and the ferry that took tourists out to explore the trails on McNabs Island.

A week earlier, Halifax hosted some of the world's top leaders for the G7 economic summit. In preparation for the media blitz, the city gave the waterfront a facelift, and a newly created area of boardwalk called "Summit Plaza" extended south of the main tourist areas. This was the direction we headed. Away from the mobs of summer tourists lingering over dinner and drinks on the outdoor restaurant patios. My dad had never been a fan of crowds.

I hooked my arm in Dad's and walked with him beside the water. We didn't talk right away. When there was a lot to say, our habit was to say nothing. The evening was chilly. I was glad for the light sweater I'd slipped on before leaving the house. I breathed in the salty, ocean air. Mom and Chris walked ahead, chatting about the new boardwalk construction.

Dad's gait was a bit off balance, and, within a few minutes, his breath was labored. I slowed my pace and stopped next to a bench that faced the water. I pointed to a large sailboat with towering double masts that motored out past the mouth of the harbor. "Is that the *Bluenose?*" I asked. The restored vessel was a replica of a historic racing schooner from the 1920s. Its iconic image adorned Nova Scotia's license plates and Canada's dime. For years it had provided chartered tours of the Halifax Harbor, but it hadn't been around for the last couple of summers.

"They repaired its hull and launched it again just in time for the summit," Dad said, resting his hand on the bench for support. Chris and Mom circled back to where we stood. "It was quite something to see the news feature Bill Clinton, Jacques Chirac, and the other leaders taking a cruise." A wistfulness filled Dad's eyes as he watched the billowing white sails climb slowly up the masts.

He was a boat guy. For many summers of my childhood, our motor-boat, the *Mainstay*, provided endless recreation. When Dad and Mom moved to Halifax, they purchased a used, seventeen-foot sailboat: *The Songstress*. They moored it in a picturesque inlet called Hubbards Cove, about forty minutes from Halifax. Weekends on the water soothed them into coping with the fresh realities of Dad's progressing illness and gave them their own mooring as they settled into their new life chapter in Nova Scotia. For the last four summers, sailing was a central family activity when any of us were home, and I developed an abiding love for the quiet calm of skimming through water under nature's power.

At the end of last summer, without any conversation or fanfare, Dad sold *The Songstress.* An intuition, perhaps, warned him he would not have the strength to keep sailing for another season. I knew it broke his heart. I also knew he did it for my mother. He was subtly unsaddling her from anything that might be a burden after he died.

When the 143-foot *Bluenose* was under full sails, she was a spectacular sight. The black sheen of her wooden hull against the white canvas gracing her masts was beautiful. I continued to hold Dad's arm, and we watched the ship glide along the water. The other sailboats and powerboats drifting in the harbor looked tiny in comparison.

After a few minutes, Dad sat down on the bench. "Well, Dorsie," he said looking to where my mother stood. "I think you'd better take me back."

"Feeling okay?" she asked, sitting down beside him.

"Just a little tired," he said. A look passed between them, and I wondered if "tired" was code for something more. "You guys should keep walking, though," he said, looking at Chris and me. "The new boardwalk is really pretty the farther down you go, and it's such a nice evening."

"We will," I promised. I didn't ask if he wanted us to come back with them to the hospital. I knew he didn't.

"I'll call in the morning," Dad said as he stood up. He gave me a quick smile and added, "We'll discuss another 'expedition,' and Dave needs our input on his valedictory speech."

"See you at home," Mom said and reached for Dad's hand.

They turned and walked slowly back the way we'd come, their hands intertwined. This was the only way I knew my parents, the only way I could imagine them. As one complete unit. My eyes burned as I watched the distance between us widen.

Chris took my hand and pulled me toward the newly constructed path next to the water. "Let's walk, Mellie," he said. I gripped his fingers and reluctantly turned away from the direction my parents had gone.

The Dress Rehearsal

I BRUSHED AWAY tears as anger surged up my spine. I wanted to kick something or someone, but I was fixed to this spot, outside my parents' bedroom in the upstairs hallway of their Halifax home, staring at the paneled door that my brother Mark had just shut behind me, cutting me off from Dad. I hadn't protested what was happening as it happened, and now, there was no one to protest to. I was the only one out here.

Mike, Mark, David, and Mom were still in the bedroom. I heard their muffled voices and movements on the other side of the door. They all had something to do, a role to play, in this practical moment of care for my potentially dying father.

I did not.

This message was delivered loudly and clearly with the shutting of the bedroom door. My anger dissipated into the stifling air of the hallway. "It's not fair," I whispered to no one. Dejection stepped in.

I'd never felt so useless.

It was the first week of August, and apprehension rode the air like an electric charge. Dad was sick. So sick, in fact, that Mom had called the family home. A week ago, Chris and I drove to Halifax under a cloud of anxiety, our vacation in Pennsylvania with my in-laws cut short. Michael and Yvonne flew in a day later from Toronto. David still lived at home but was making preparations to leave for his first year of college. Though Mark had an apartment of his own downtown near the children's hospital where he was finishing up his second year of residency, for the past couple of days he had camped out with the rest of us at the house.

"It's called pneumocystis pneumonia, or PCP," Mark explained on my first day home as I sat at the foot of the bed, staring at Dad, shocked at the weakness of his form. My hand rested on his calf, the thick, down comforter separating my skin from his. Even so, I felt the heat of his fever on my fingers. Six weeks earlier, after David's high school graduation, Dad had surgery to remove his gallbladder to alleviate the stomach issues that had landed him in the hospital before our visit. Chris and I had to leave Halifax for our friends Sherri and Tim's wedding in Ottawa—Chris was the best man, and I was the matron of honor. After the wedding when all signs pointed to a good recovery for Dad, we returned to Baltimore for a week and then continued with our plans to spend a few weeks with Chris's parents at the family farm that was their summer home. This new infection came out of nowhere and hit Dad hard.

Despite efforts to keep the bedroom dim, afternoon sun leaked through the cotton drapes drawn across the patio doors. A pleasant breeze drifted past the open screens, and the curtain fabric fluttered across the carpeted floor. The bag of clear liquid hanging at the top of the IV pole next to the bed caught the light and reflected it in shards onto the wall above the headboard.

Dad was sleeping comfortably as far as I could tell, but the pallor of his skin, his labored breathing, the wheeze in his lungs, audible above the hum of the portable machine that fed oxygen through a tube in his nostrils, spoke to a definitive shift in his health since I last saw him.

"It's what we call an 'opportunistic infection' because it takes advantage of someone with a compromised immune system, like Dad," Mark continued. He fiddled with the IV tube as he spoke and then bent over to check the bag hanging off the side of the bed that I knew attached to Dad's catheter.

"So, what does that really mean?" I asked, wishing I understood the science of this mystifying disease. I relied on Mark to sidestep the euphemistic language my mother used to keep me from worrying and tell me the truth. Most of the time he was good about it.

"It means we have to wait," he said with a sigh, leaning his weight on the pine bedpost. Dark shadows under his eyes told me that being charged with the medical care to honor Dad's desire to remain at home this time wasn't easy. Mark's wedding to Ellen was only two and a half weeks away, but the joy of their preparations was snuffed out by this latest crisis. "The steroids we've given Dad to help his lung function take time to work. We have to wait and see what they do. We have to wait and see if these new antiviral meds knock down his fever. We just have to wait."

So waiting was what we'd been doing for a week. None of us was willing to call what we were doing a death vigil, but it looked and felt an awful lot like I imagined one would. During the daytime hours, we took turns sitting with Dad to make sure someone was always there when he woke up. When he did open his eyes, when he met our gaze and whispered hoarsely, "How doin'?" we all flocked to his side to savor the minutes he was with us before fatigue and the fog of meds pulled him away once more.

In each of these moments of lucidity, I was haunted by an all-too-familiar fear. A looming question that, for ten years, had attached to every holiday, every vacation, every visit, every phone call, every sign of illness.

Is this it?

I didn't know what signs to look for to answer this question, and I was too frightened to ask. Instead, I stayed with Dad as much as I could, with the hope that seeing his daughter with her gift of cheerfulness when he woke up was doing as much to help him as the meds dripping from the IV bag into the bruised vein in his arm.

Right before I was ousted to the hallway outside my parents' bedroom, I was sitting with Dad when he startled awake and said, "The bed feels damp." I called downstairs to Mark and Mom, figuring that Dad's catheter might have leaked. I picked up the glass of water from the bedside table and asked Dad if he wanted a drink. He nodded, and I held the bent straw to his lips so he could take a sip. He gave me a weak smile in thanks, and then said, "I think I wet the bed." His confession held a note of humor, but I also heard a tone of humiliation. Even at his most vulnerable, my father was a proud man.

"We'll fix it in a sec, Dad," I said. "Hold tight." I wanted to reassure him and let him know that it wasn't a big deal. I took his hand and gave it a squeeze.

Mark and Mom came in, followed by Mike and Dave. "The sheets are wet," I told them, beginning to fold back the comforter to see if it was wet too. Mark was in doctor mode. He moved to the side of the bed where the catheter line wound under the covers and lifted them.

"His cath came loose," he said to Mom. "I need to adjust it, and we'll need to change the bed and his pajamas."

Dad was too weak to sit up on his own, and I recognized that we were all needed to move him off the wet linens to get the bed changed. Mom went in search of new sheets and pajamas while I moved to the other side of the bed with David, preparing to do my part to help lift Dad.

"Mel," Mark said, authority sharpening his voice. I looked up. "Let's try and preserve Dad's dignity here," he nodded toward the door. "You should go."

Heat scalded my cheeks and resentment saturated my body. I looked at Michael and David who were not given the same instructions. Why did I have to go? Just because I'm the daughter? And not the doctor? I wasn't an idiot. I could preserve Dad's dignity without having to leave the room. I could help change the sheets. That was something in this whole fucking mess that I actually knew how to do. I even knew how to do hospital corners, from my days as a candy striper in high school. I could avert my eyes when I needed to. I was a grown woman.

But Mark pulled rank, and his command left me feeling like a reprimanded child. Instead of launching the arguments that rushed up my throat, I reverted to my accustomed role as the little sister. I was defenseless against my brother's wielded power, and I slunk out the door without speaking. He pushed it closed behind me.

Now, as I walked down the stairs farther away from the only place I wanted to be, I said the words again. "It's not fair." Even as I spoke,

I could rationalize Mark's actions. He wasn't trying to hurt me. He thought he was doing the right thing for Dad's sake. Maybe even for mine.

Except he wasn't. He had no idea what it felt like to be me in the face of Dad's illness. He didn't know what it felt like to sit and watch Dad weaken day after day and be helpless to do *anything*. He didn't know because he got to do something. Every day. I knew that balancing the role of caretaker and son must feel impossible to him. But as the rest of us sat around waiting, he got to walk into that bedroom and be the one who knew how to make Dad sleep more comfortably. Knew how to help him breathe better. Knew how to adjust his IV or fix his catheter. He knew how to take away Dad's pain. And because he knew what signs to look for, he also knew how to answer the looming question I was too scared to ask.

But he didn't know what it was like to be me while he was doing all that practical work, what it was like to feel so useless. He didn't know that when he'd snatched away my one chance to help, he'd taken something bigger from me. And I wouldn't tell him, even with the sharp sting of the separation still burning. What good would that do?

—

The burn in my calf muscles and the fresh air in my lungs felt good as I sprinted down Julie's Walk a few strides behind Chris. We passed the car-crowded driveway, slowed to a walk, and drew in deep breaths. Five other houses besides my parents' sat on this quaint cul-de-sac. I looked toward the upstairs dormer window. The blinds that had been closed for days were still closed. Sweat beaded on my forehead and ran down the sides of my face. With my hands resting on my hips, I circled the street a few times to bring down my heart rate. Chris matched my gait and ran his fingers through his damp hair. We didn't speak. We'd talked ourselves out for the last four miles. I wanted to stay outside a little longer and feel the late morning sun on my skin while I pretended everything was okay. My eyes returned to the upstairs window.

Everything was not okay.

The status of Dad's pneumocystis pneumonia had not improved, and he was not responding to meds. He was besieged by an endless fatigue and unable to get out of bed. He couldn't breathe without oxygen, and his body was getting weaker. There was now quiet talk of postponing Mark and Ellen's wedding. Dad could be dying.

The waiting for confirmation of this fact one way or another was agony.

Each day melted into the next with little change and little for any of us to do. When Dad was awake, which was not often, we took turns keeping him company, trying not to exhaust him with too much commotion. A few days earlier, my sister-in-law Yvonne had gone out and gotten some craft materials, and she and I had spent hours painting terra cotta flowerpots on the back deck. I have little artistic talent and my pots could have been mistaken for a child's grade school project, but I was grateful for something that kept my hands busy and distracted my mind.

Running was another respite. The daily ritual provided an escape from the leaden uneasiness that filled every crevice of the house. This morning, Chris and I had woven through the hilly streets of my parents' neighborhood, pushing our bodies hard, relishing the chance to focus on something solid: movement from point A to point B. Looping the cul-de-sac, I savored the fleeting high of the endorphins coursing through my system.

As we circled back toward the house, a neighbor walked down his shrub-lined driveway toward us, wheeling his bicycle beside him. I didn't know him well. I didn't know any of the neighbors well. Mom and Dad had moved to this house when I left for college, and though I came home every summer and lived at home for a year of graduate school before Chris and I got married, there weren't many opportunities to interact. Everyone on this street did a good job of keeping to themselves. This man was some sort of software engineer and worked from home. Most of his work appeared to involve tinkering with the thirty-foot sailboat parked in his driveway. He was married with two young kids and an old, blind Cocker Spaniel that liked to pee on my parents' front lawn, leaving dead, yellow patches in the grass. My dad vowed to plant a stake in the neighbor's yard with a stern note expressing his displeasure at the dog's behavior. My mother talked him out of it.

"Good day for a run," the neighbor said, stopping in the street beside us, noting our sweat-soaked running clothes.

"It is," I said. I was in no mood for small talk, especially with someone I'd never talked to before.

"How's your dad? We heard he'd taken a bad turn." He looked pointedly at the extra cars in the driveway and lining the curb in front of my parents' house. I was caught off guard. Even though Dad's HIV status had become common knowledge with the publication of The Book a few months earlier, I'd been too far away to be part of the big reveal or to receive the responses of support from friends and strangers near and far. I was startled to be confronted with overt questions about Dad's health and talking about it without restriction felt new and strange.

"He's not doing very well," Chris answered for me. I threw him a grateful look.

"Aw, shit," the neighbor said, shaking his head. "I figured as much when I saw the out-of-province license plates." He leaned on the handlebars of his bike and tilted his head toward the sky. "God, it's so awful. I can't stop thinking about it." His voice shook a little.

"Yeah," I said, unsure how to respond. His eyes turned back to me and probed mine until I had to look away. I sensed he was hoping for comfort. I had none to give.

He swept his hand across his forehead. "I'm all fucked up about it. All. Fucked. Up."

"Yeah," I said again like this was a perfectly normal conversation to be having with a stranger. We stood, quiet and awkward, and I stared at the scuffed toes of my sneakers. Chris cleared his throat. The neighbor didn't move. I now understood that this guy was going to stay there expounding on his fucked-upness unless I took the initiative and moved things along. "Well, I guess we should probably get back," I said.

All Fucked Up (forever thereafter known only in my family as AFU) straightened his shoulders and swung his leg over his bicycle. "Right, right." He looked past me to the house, as though staring hard enough might allow him to see inside. "You take care," he said. "Take good care," he repeated. He settled on the bike seat and clipped his feet into the pedals. "Tell your dad we're thinking of him and praying for the best."

"I will. Thanks," I said and watched him ride up the street. He disappeared around the corner, and I turned back to Chris. We both started laughing, but even after Chris had laughed himself out, I couldn't stop. I doubled over, gasping with tears streaming down my cheeks. The knots in my chest loosened with each labored breath. The release felt good.

When I was able to speak, I looked at Chris and said, "Seriously? *He's* all fucked up?"

The Rally

I STOOD WITH the other members of the wedding party in the vestibule of St. Andrew's United Church in Mirimachi, New Brunswick, waiting for my turn to process down the aisle. Dressed in a gorgeous white raw silk gown, her expression hidden by a misty veil, Ellen waited a few feet behind me, her arm linked with her father's. In one hand I clutched the tight bouquet of pink, peach, and cream roses against the white lace top I wore and with the other I smoothed the front of my coral silk skirt. The rich notes of the processional floated from the organ, and I watched my mother's careful walk, her hand gripping Mark's arm, to the front pew of the church where my sister-in-law Yvonne already sat. At their approach, a side door opened and Chris appeared, handsome in a dark suit, his head slightly bent, pushing my dad's wheelchair in front of him. Dad sat straight in the chair, but the stiff line of his neck and shoulders betrayed the effort of the exertion. His eyes were trained straight ahead, and his face was fixed with a tight smile. At the lip of the door's threshold, a wheel caught and stalled their forward progress for a moment, and Dad's smile faltered, but Chris managed to back up and then maneuver the chair and guide it across the front of the sanctuary to meet Mom at her seat. As Mark took his place next to his line of groomsmen and Mom sat down, Chris positioned Dad's chair next to her. He locked the brakes, removed the portable oxygen tank that Dad balanced on his lap and set it at his side. He straightened a long plastic tube that attached to the tank and wound up to the clear nasal cannula that looped over Dad's ears and stretched across his face. Chris stepped past my mother and took his seat next to Yvonne. As he sat down, his body relaxed.

I released the breath I'd been holding for the maybe twenty seconds the whole procedure had taken and blinked back tears that threatened to spill down my cheeks. Nobody in that sanctuary would question the reason I might be crying as I walked down the aisle—the miracle of Dad's presence in this moment, after he'd come frighteningly close to death only weeks before, was not lost on anyone—but it was critically important to Dad that his illness not cast shade on the joy of this day.

Two weeks ago, Mark and Ellen were making plans to postpone their wedding when, to everyone's surprise, Dad's health took a turn for the better after a last desperate effort to fight off the pneumonia with a high-intensity round of new IV antibiotics. His fever broke. He became more lucid, started eating again, and the color returned to his skin. He regained some strength and could sit up for short periods at a time. However, he was still plagued by fatigue and slept for large portions of the day. His lungs depended on supplemental oxygen. This rebound felt transient and fragile. Dr. Marrie, Dad's doctor, who'd been making house calls during the crisis and knew all of the stakes, was not in favor of him trying to make the four-hour trip for the wedding from my parents' home in Halifax to Ellen's hometown of Mirimachi. "The stress of the drive alone could kill you," he told my father. Making the wedding happen with Dad there seemed an unworkable endeavor.

And then a family friend made a generous offer. He owned a luxury RV equipped with all of the comforts of home, including a spacious bedroom with a king-sized bed. What if he drove my dad and mom to and from Mirimachi? Dad could sleep the entire way, they could drive straight through without having to stop at any public rest areas where Dad's compromised immune system might be exposed to infection, and he wouldn't risk overworking his weakened lungs. This arrangement was enough to convince Dr. Marrie to let Dad go, as long as he adhered to stern guidelines for limiting his activity during the weekend festivities to the rehearsal, the actual ceremony, and the early part of the reception, and used a wheelchair at all times.

The wheelchair was a blow to Dad's ego. The show of having to be wheeled down the church aisle, his portable oxygen tank in tow, at the center of everyone's gaze, was his nightmare scenario. When we'd returned after wedding rehearsal the day before to the hotel room where he was resting, propped up against a stack of fluffy pillows, and informed him of the church set up, he'd latched onto the alternative of making an inconspicuous entrance in his wheelchair through the side door at the front of the sanctuary.

"I want it to be Chris," Dad said when Michael and David started volleying the logistics of how one of them would wheel him in and then join the rest of the groomsmen. "I want Chris to push me in." He turned to where my husband sat in a chair near the bed. "That okay with you?"

"Yes sir," Chris said easily.

"Okay then. It's settled," Dad said, and the conversation shifted to how many cars we should take to the rehearsal dinner so that Mom and Dad would be able to bow out when he got tired. From where I sat at the foot of the bed, I reached for Chris's hand. Something big had just happened, but I might have been the only one who noticed.

Chris and I met on my first day at Gordon College in 1990. He was a sophomore and a member of the orientation staff. The orientation committee was throwing an ice cream social for the new students, and he was standing behind one of many tables lined up in the large gymnasium, wearing a stained apron and scooping chocolate ice cream from a huge vat into Styrofoam bowls. "You're Michael's sister, right?" he asked when I approached and reached for a bowl. "I'm Chris Brooks." He smiled and put out his hand, and I took it. His fingers were sticky, but his grip was strong. After a dizzying day of moving into my dorm room, saying a tearful goodbye to my mother, and trying to acclimate to my new surroundings, his steadiness felt like something I wanted to hold onto. That he was a familiar name in this crowd of strangers helped too. My brother had graduated that spring with a major in economics and a minor in music, and Chris's parents—both music professors at the college—had basically adopted him into their family in his last two years there. When I decided to follow in my brother's collegiate footsteps, Mike urged me to connect with the Brookses, letting me know that they were among the few people he'd confided in about Dad's health.

Over the following week, Chris and I bumped into each other a few more times, and after two weeks, he asked me out. As I got to know him better, I was drawn to his authenticity and warmth. With three gregarious older brothers and a father like mine, I was not accustomed to Chris's way of being in the world—confident enough to steer clear of the spotlight at social gatherings and not out to impress anybody, thoughtful and observant, dependable and even-tempered, comfortable with quiet and slow to enter a conversation—but it put me at ease. That he knew my biggest secret without me having to tell him made him someone who knew *me*. And the relief of being known allowed me to open up to him in ways I'd never done with anyone else.

We dated for the next three years. For everyone who knew us in our day-to-day lives at school, we were a solid match—a perfect blend of personality traits and obviously devoted to each other based on the strength and longevity of our relationship. Unfortunately, my parents were not among those people. For most of those three years, they were disconnected from our growing relationship. They lived eleven hours away, and though Chris visited with us in Nova Scotia for a week or two during the summer and for a few days at the holidays, they didn't get to know him as I knew him. And because he wasn't like what they were accustomed to either, he wasn't an easy sell.

"He seems a little quiet," my mother said after their first meeting.

My father wasn't as delicate with his take. "What's he going to do with a history major? Are you sure he's not just boring?"

I can't imagine what it was like for my father to live with the ever-present knowledge that he wasn't going to be around to make sure his children's lives turned out okay. What I do know is that my brothers and I lived under the pressure of his fears, stretched at the seams to please him. He was preoccupied about helping us plan for our futures. He scrutinized our decisions with an intensity that bordered on obsessive, including our choice of partners.

Even without the boundaries created by Dad's health situation, our family was not an easy one to break into. Exceptional was the established status quo. The Messenger Way—effusive responses to pretty much everything, exhibition of talents on demand, endless competitive play and banter, and well-defined, ambitious plans for future success (preferably ones that involved a professional degree)—was not Chris's way. He was nine years older than his one brother so never had to vie for position in his family. His parents were both professional performers—his mother a former opera singer and his father a choral conductor—and while they'd inhabited center-stage, Chris had grown up in the wings. In contrast to my idyllic childhood summers with family at a secluded cottage on a coastal river, he spent many of those summers with his eccentric grandparents on their farm in Pennsylvania while his parents toured Europe for weeks at a time. He'd learned how to be comfortable being alone. My family dynamics suffocated him sometimes and made him turn inward. Acutely in tune with their responses, I feared my parents read his distance as disinterestedness.

"Can't you just be a little more outgoing? A little more like my brothers?" I pleaded with him during a visit, one of the only times when I ever felt my confidence in my feelings for Chris waver as it battled against my need for my family's, specifically my father's, approval.

"This is me, Mel," he sighed, not hiding the hurt in his voice. "I can't be someone I'm not."

It took getting away from the force of my family's expectations to solidify my feelings that Chris was exactly the partner I wanted him to be. To understand that being with him made me better. I wrapped my arms around this one radical act of rebellion and instead of waiting for my dad's approval, I allowed myself to trust my own instincts. A month after graduation, Chris and I got engaged.

Even though he helped us with the wedding plans and made an effort to welcome Chris into our family, Dad didn't hide his enduring doubts, patriarchal as they were, about what kind of future Chris might be able to provide for me. "How will a master's degree in Medieval European History lead to a stable life for my daughter?" he'd asked Chris outright not long after our engagement. As someone who'd known his own career trajectory from age fifteen, accepting Chris's plans to pursue this graduate degree without a clear picture of the end game was tough. Dad's fears made it tough for me too. I wanted to reassure him, and I wished he could believe in Chris the way I did. I didn't have to see the future etched in stone to know that we'd be okay wherever we ended up. I just worried that my dad wouldn't be with us long enough to know it too.

But then Dad asked Chris to push his wheelchair into the sanctuary on Mark and Ellen's wedding day. As I watched Dad and Chris's brief journey from side door to pew, the tears that threatened to undo all of my careful makeup held much more than gratitude that my father was still alive. I could read the vulnerability in Dad's sunken eyes, could see how off-balance this whole situation made him feel. And I understood that choosing my husband for this task was Dad's way of showing me that the steadiness I felt the first time I took Chris's ice-cream covered hand in mine was something Dad, too, wanted to hold.

HEAVY

That time
I thought I could not
go any closer to grief
without dying

I went closer,
and I did not die.

MARY OLIVER,
"Heavy"

Not the Most Wonderful Time of the Year

2013

THE SMELL OF ground coffee beans and the murmur of small talk filled the space as I stood in line inside the crowded Starbucks a few miles from my home.

"Can I get something started for you, hon?" the cheerful, thick-necked guy behind the counter asked when he caught my eye. A white bandana wrapped around his head and covered the top half of a mop of shoulder-length curls. I chose not to question the bandana's effective-ness nor be offended at his use of "hon," since he was the link to my much-needed caffeine fix of the morning.

"Venti Earl Grey tea, one tea bag, with room for milk," I said.

"Anything to eat with that?" he asked as I handed him my credit card. My eyes swept the glass case to my right. Giant muffins with crumbled toppings, flaky pastries, chocolate-covered squares, oversized cookies, those cake pops covered in colorful sprinkles—they all looked deli-cious. And fattening.

"No, thanks." I held my resolve. "Just the tea."

I stood to the side and waited for my drink. A tall man in a neatly pressed black suit stepped up to the counter and gave another barista a complex coffee order that included the words "red eye" and "two shots of espresso." He was the kind of Starbucks patron who made me feel subpar. My standard tea was dull in comparison to the array of coffee drinks on the menu. I loved the smell of coffee, but the only way I could stomach the bitter taste was to infuse it with cream and enough sugar to make it like ice cream.

"Here you go, hon," Bandana Guy said and passed me my cup.

I brushed past Mr. Red Eye and the other customers in line and headed toward the small bar with the insulated pitchers of cream and milk and small square boxes overflowing with packets of sugar and sweeteners. It was only when I started to pour the skim milk into my tea that I noticed the bright red cup for the first time. Images traced in gold floated across its surface: poinsettias, ornaments of various shapes and sizes, symmetrical snowflakes.

"You've got to be kidding me," I said.

It was November 4th. The trees were making that shift from the October peaks of red, orange, and yellow to the rusted, earthy tones that signaled late fall. I was still basking in the glow of mothering success I had achieved with the handmade *Despicable Me* minion Halloween costume I'd labored over for Lily the week before. On the counter in my kitchen, covered in Saran Wrap, sat two remaining pieces of the round, homemade jack-o-lantern chocolate cake. Earlier that morning, I had posted my mid-term warning grades for my college students. Christmas was nowhere on my radar.

Until now.

Bandana Guy handed me a decorated Starbucks cup, and the holidays were here. Apprehension stretched across my shoulders and threaded into my chest. Too soon, I thought. I am not ready.

I looked at the other customers who milled about Starbucks and sipped from their festive, seasonal cups. Was I the only one who felt blindsided by this sudden reminder of the approaching holiday season? Was I the only one who struggled to balance the joy I was *supposed* to be feeling with the dread I was *actually* feeling? Was I the only one who wanted to yell: Can we just slow things down for a second?

Going Closer

LARGE SNOWFLAKES DOTTED the backdrop outside, and a light dusting of white was beginning to stick to the ground and the trees visible through the window over Dr. B's shoulder. It was early December, and the air was cold, but we hadn't had a significant snowfall yet. The forecast predicted this one might materialize into something meaningful.

"I love the first snow of the season," I said, watching the accumulating flakes.

"Me too," Dr. B said and turned in his chair to look out the window. "It's so clean."

"There's something comforting and peaceful about it," I said and then sighed. "I wish it would all just stay that way."

Dr. B turned back to me. "How are things this week?" he asked. The question and the probing look in his eyes told me he knew the "all" that I wished would stay peaceful reached beyond the snowy landscape.

"I guess I'm okay," I said and noted my unconvincing choice of words. Why did I think I needed Dr. B to go through the extra effort of peeling back the layers of meaning here to get to my actual feelings? It was the same tactic I used on everyone: show me you care, and maybe I'll tell you the truth. It seemed like my therapist should be exempt from the task. So, I threw him a lifeline. "My mom called me in the middle of the afternoon yesterday."

Dr. B listened and waited for me to continue.

"I can always predict that when she calls on a weekday when I might be teaching, that she's got something bothering her."

"And did she?" Dr. B asked.

I nodded and gave him the recap.

When the house phone in the kitchen jangled the day before, I ignored it and continued reading the part in my student Peter's short story where his main character is confronted with scenes from his past at the instant of his death. Peter had used quick flashbacks to weave in the important backstory that was missing when we'd workshopped the piece the first time around. *Wahoo!* I typed, my fingers flying across my laptop keyboard. *Suddenly Charles is a character we can invest in because you've helped us to get to know him better, Peter!*

I shifted my weight in the red club chair. The sun shone through the picture windows in the living room and shed slanted sunbeams across the hardwood floor. Wally, our Lab, had found one and slept next to my chair, his yellow head resting on his paws. I'd been sitting in the same position for almost three hours, determined to read as many writing portfolios as I could before Will and Lily came home from school. I'd promised my creative writing students at Nashua Community College that I'd have their grades for our final class on Friday. Christmas was less than three weeks away, and, since its arrival in this house depended in large part on me, I needed to get this task off of my plate.

My cell phone vibrated on the coffee table in front of me. Wally startled at the sound and stood, opening his mouth in a wide yawn. I reached for the phone and read the ID on the screen: *Mom.*

The phone buzzed again. It had been a few days since I'd talked to my mother, and I welcomed a break from my grading. My shoulders ached. I pushed the answer button. "Hi," I said, shutting my laptop and leaning back in my chair.

"What are you doing?" Mom's voice sounded unnaturally bright.

"Just some grading. What's going on there?" I scratched Wally's ears, and he settled back in his spot on the floor.

"Well, I'm putting out all of my Christmas decorations, and it's making me very sad," she said in a breathless rush. "I just needed to hear your voice." Sorrow attached to the final statement.

"Oh, Mom," I said and felt my own sorrow sneaking in. "Are you doing it all by yourself? Where's John?"

"He's out running an errand. You know he wouldn't be interested in this anyway," she said. Resentment sharpened her voice. I clamped down hard on my back teeth, the muscles in my jaw tight.

My mother's husband was a self-proclaimed Scrooge. He wasn't much for celebrating anything, and he didn't care about what he perceived as the trappings of the Christmas season. "Why bother about a tree?" he'd stunned Mom by asking the first Christmas after their wedding. His anti-joy campaign failed to deter her, though. She insisted on decking the halls of their home despite his indifference. Christmas traditions mattered to my mother.

I fixed my eyes on the twinkling tree in the corner of our living room. The night before, with Bing Crosby crooning favorite carols in the background, we'd finished our own decorating. The porcelain-faced angel that topped the seven-foot Fraser fir grazed the ceiling, and the tree's boughs displayed a varied collection of ornaments. Scattered among the ones Chris and I had accumulated in the two decades we'd been married were the keepsakes my parents had given me from the time I was a little girl. We'd carried on the tradition with Will and Lily. Every year, we presented each with a new ornament. Their childhoods were chronicled on the fragrant evergreen branches. Buzz Lightyear and Batman. Dora the Explorer and a pink tutued ballerina. Soccer balls and baseball gloves. Basketball players and gymnasts. A Red Sox Nutcracker, a Patriots Santa, a Bruins Snowman, a Celtics jersey. A yellow Lab wearing a Santa hat marked Wally's entrance to our family the previous year. The newest ornaments: the 2013 World Series commemorative balls for both kids—Will's red, Lily's navy blue.

I wished I could bridge the physical distance between Mom and me to offer her some comfort, and I tried to keep my own long-standing resentment about John's lack of interest in what was important to her at bay. "I'm so sorry, Mom," I said. My words felt hollow. Insufficient.

"Every little thing I take out of the box brings back so many memories," she said. "So many reminders of Dad. The little mouse carolers holding their songbooks. I just set up the old nativity. The one from Grammie Messenger's house. Remember that?"

"Mm hmm," I said. Of course, I did. I closed my eyes and saw Dad and me leaning over the flat cardboard base. Patiently, he helped me sound out the words to the labeled tabs where the lithographed figures could be inserted to stand upright. *Place colored wise man here*, one read, a hint to the set's 1940s origin. I loved organizing the characters and putting them in the designated spots: the kneeling shepherds, the sheep and goats, the three wise men and their camels. Mary, Joseph, and the baby Jesus, their glowing halos crowning their heads. We saved the bright, yellow star for last. Dad's large hands circled mine, and together we pushed it into the grooves on top of the stable and then stood back to admire our work. Even as a little girl, I sensed something sacred in the finished scene. The magic of the very first Christmas. It didn't occur to me then that Christmas could be anything but magical.

"I just wish I lived closer to you all." Mom sighed into the phone.

I heard the loneliness in her voice. I wished she lived closer too. My heart hurt as I pictured her sitting alone in front of a stack of Rubbermaid bins, pulling out familiar decorations and trying to decide where they should go.

This was not how things were supposed to be.

"I'm just being silly," she said.

Now I sighed. I recognized where this conversation was headed. The same direction most of the conversations about the pain of our loss headed in my family: as far away from the pain as possible.

"Mom, it's not silly," I said. "You're allowed to be sad."

"Oh, I know," she said, her voice over-bright again. "But what can you do? We just have to get on with things." There it was. The Messenger Family Code of Survival. The fundamental rules? Carry on. Don't dwell.

Across the street, my neighbor's diesel pickup idled in his driveway, its engine roar harsh against the quiet of midday.

"You are allowed to be sad, Mom," I said again. I put some added force behind my words. They were important for me to hear too. Therapy had emboldened me to say them out loud. My father died senselessly and way too soon. And he died at Christmas.

The experience demanded dwelling.

"I started feeling it yesterday sitting in church. Hearing the carols. It's just the week, you know?" Mom said, the emotion returning to her voice.

I did know. A subtle cloud of melancholy always accompanied the arrival of Christmas and settled over me like a shroud. I'd felt its presence as soon as the Starbucks barista handed me that holiday cup. This Friday—December 13th—would mark eighteen years since Dad died. Though I loved the season's white lights and flickering candles, the fragrant garlands and colorful bows, the familiar carols and longstanding traditions, they also framed the moment of my deepest sorrow and served as aching reminders. I'd been struggling to cope with my sadness for days—overstretched by the tension of wanting to create Christmas joy for my family and wishing I could escape it all.

"This week is hard, Mom," I said. "It always is." I longed for her to ask me how I was doing. How I was feeling. To invite me to bring my grief into the conversation. Would I even tell her if she did? I was well-practiced at stuffing my pain out of sight, excellent at deflecting. Easier than having it dismissed. Or rushed, which my mother was sometimes prone to do.

"No use being sad by myself," Mom said. "I just need to stop thinking about it." I held the phone tighter. She wouldn't be asking me how I was doing.

I rested my free hand on Wally's back, soothed by the softness of his fur. He lifted his head and looked at me with his questioning brown eyes before pushing his body into my touch. "Is John sympathetic at all?" I asked Mom.

"Oh, he doesn't really know about any of it," she said. "I don't talk about that stuff with him."

A new wave of sadness joined the already churning sea in my gut. Genuine closeness was absent from my mother's marriage to John. The things that had appealed to her when they'd met—his interest, like hers, in fitness; the idea of someone to fill the loneliness— were not a strong enough foundation to build on. Their daily interactions revolved around only what was on the surface: the activity of their day, headlines in the newspaper, crosswords, the latest Red Sox score. The comfortable familiarity that develops over time in most relationships just wasn't there. Almost eight years in, they still wandered around each other like strangers. I suspected my mom was lonely in the relationship, and no safe space existed for her to share these feelings, this grief—some of the most defining pieces of who she was.

My mind traveled to the previous night, when I'd sobbed my sadness against Chris's chest in the darkness of our bedroom. The complete security in that moment of intimacy gave me permission to loosen the hold I kept on my emotions at all other times. Chris was my safe space.

"I'm all right. Really," Mom said. She was backpedaling. Making light. She'd opened the door on her pain, and now she was pushing it closed again. I kept my foot in just a crack.

"Of course you're not all right," I said. "How could you be? Those ornaments? Those decorations? They represent what went unfinished. The future that didn't happen the way you and Dad planned when you got them. You can be sad for longer than a few minutes about that."

"That's hard to do when you are around someone who doesn't understand," she said. Her voice was weary. "I can only be sad in my head."

I bit my lip. The same questions I'd been asking for years pushed against it. Why wouldn't he understand? He lost his wife too. Why don't you try to talk to him about what you are feeling? The only way he can know is if you tell him. Why stay with someone who can't or won't share your pain? Why did you marry him in the first place? Whatever the litany beforehand, it always ended on that question.

These were old laments with no satisfactory answers. "John knows he's not your first husband, Mom," I said instead. "He has to understand that you'd grieve for what came before—especially this week. It's a hard week."

"It is," she conceded.

We were both quiet for a minute, lost in our shared memories.

She sighed once more and said, "I think I hear John."

"You can still be sad, Mom."

"Thanks, honey," her voice changed. Bright once more. She closed the door and returned to the pleasantries. "Oh, I think John and I might drive out to Kennetcook on Friday," she said. I heard murmuring in the background. John's voice adding something to the conversation. "It all depends on the weather. John says there might be snow."

My teeth clenched tighter. I loathed the idea of John being anywhere near the picturesque country churchyard where my dad was buried. Where we'd buried my Grammie Messenger eight months after Dad died, in the plot next to his dad, the grandfather I'd never met. I knew I wasn't being fair to John, but I hated it anyway. To me, that place was hallowed ground. He did not belong.

"I'll take pictures and text them," Mom added. She typically did this when she made the yearly pilgrimage to the cemetery in a sincere effort to include us in the journey. I didn't say that I was not sure I could bear another wrenching snapshot of her squatting next to Dad's headstone in the snow, her hand lightly resting on the black granite.

"Okay," I said.

"Well, dear, I'll let you get back to your marking," Mom said. "Thanks for the chat."

"Are you really okay?" I asked.

"Oh yes. Fine. Don't you worry, okay? I love you."

"I love you, too, Mom," I said and tapped the end button on the screen. The phone felt heavy in my hand. Everything felt heavy.

I stared out the window. The blue of the sky seemed deeper. Darker. Shapeless clouds drifted over its surface. My neighbor's truck was gone, and the street was now quiet. A fat squirrel sat motionless on a bare branch of the dogwood tree near the driveway.

Longing stabbed my chest. I rested my hand over the spot beneath my collarbone, an attempt to stifle the ache that pressed out from the inside. I didn't want to pick up my laptop and go back to grading the rest of the portfolios. My momentum waned. My earlier enthusiasm zapped. I felt sluggish, like a deflated balloon. I leaned my head back against the chair and closed my eyes.

I did the same thing now as I finished telling Dr. B about the phone call. I didn't open my eyes when I whispered, "I miss my dad."

Dr. B allowed the assertion to settle in with us.

"Of course, you do," he eventually said. "There are so many reminders at this time of year, especially."

I opened my eyes and sat straighter. "Every year, as Death Day approaches, I tell myself, 'It's just a day. A day like any other day.' And I try to pretend it's no big deal. But every year, when it arrives, it flattens me."

"Maybe you shouldn't work so hard to normalize it," Dr. B mused. "Maybe that's part of the problem. It's not just a day. It's the anniversary of one of the hardest, most painful days of your life. You don't have to turn away from the difficult reality of what happened just because your mother does. I think you need to mark the day with intentionality, and I think you need to dwell in it for a while."

I thought of those dreary winter weeks after Dad died, when I'd sat in my classroom, unable to move, unable to breathe, and Mom taught me to disconnect from the sorrow, cordon it off. I might have learned too well.

Dr. B's words gave me an alternative lesson. For all these years, I'd turned away from my grief, never allowing myself to be entirely in it. I needed to go closer. To honor that melancholic cloud that descended as the holiday season approached and to also honor the reason it was there.

"I need to give myself permission to dwell," I said, trying on Dr. B's suggestion.

He pressed his palms together. "You need to give yourself permission to dwell."

The Opening Act
1995

"WHAT IS THE purpose of your visit?" the uniformed customs agent asked after scrutinizing my Canadian passport photo and then staring at me. He was handsome, his olive skin and dark hair contrasting with his light eyes. Mid-thirties, I guessed.

I tucked a loose strand of hair behind my ear and shifted my leather schoolbag on my shoulder as answers to his question catapulted through my mind: To see for myself. To see Dad for myself. To see Dad for myself and confirm what I already know is happening. Instead, I replied, "Visiting family."

My voice sounded too loud in the eerie stillness of this section of the Halifax Airport. I was one of about eight passengers from my flight passing through customs. Ours was one of those small express prop planes that seated only about thirty people, and at noon on this Saturday in late November, it hadn't been full. No other planes had arrived with ours, so besides the sole agent and a beefy security guard, we were the only ones here. This sprawling area designated for international arrivals, with its snaking queue of rows divided by stanchions and retractable belts, seemed too big a space.

I'd left behind an entirely different scene at Logan Airport in Boston earlier that day. When Chris dropped me at the curb with a peck on the cheek and a quick hug at eight that morning, the automatic doors opened to a terminal already buzzing with early Thanksgiving travelers. Ticket lines teemed with families headed all over the country to spend the holiday week with loved ones. Christmas carols sang from the sound system in between flight announcements.

At the security checkpoint to enter the departures area, I stood behind a woman who carried two huge Macy's shopping bags filled with ornately wrapped gifts. The bags were too big to fit through the X-ray machine, and she had to unload them in a flustered rush and send the presents down the conveyor belt one by one. "Got my act together early to save on postage," she said to me in explanation, though I hadn't asked. Her lipsticked mouth broke into a smile. "I'm usually not this organized." I nodded and turned away, pretending to dig for my boarding pass in my purse even though I could see it in the side pocket. I couldn't summon the energy necessary for small talk.

I was relieved to escape the chaos and crowds and buckle into my seat on the plane. No one sat next to me, so I spent the hour and a half in the air grading my tenth-grade Social Studies students' quizzes on the delegates to the Constitutional Convention and decompressing from the sensory overload of the holiday crush. Thanksgiving in Canada is celebrated on the second Monday in October, so the upcoming week held no special significance to most people on this side of the border.

"And how long will you be in Canada?" the agent asked, typing something into his computer.

"Just until Wednesday," I said. I'd cross back over to the US in time for Thanksgiving there.

I'd decided to fly to Halifax only two days earlier. I hadn't been home since Mark and Ellen's wedding in August, and even though he'd been well enough to take a trip with Mom to Barbados in October, the surge in Dad's health was short-lived.

By all accounts, he'd grown dramatically weaker in the past few weeks. These days, it sounded like the fatigue was fully debilitating. That Dr. Marrie was now exclusively making house calls spoke volumes about how hard getting out of bed must be for Dad. He needed constant oxygen to breathe. In the past two weeks, a visiting palliative care nurse had started coming weekly to monitor meds.

I called almost every day for updates, but from my spot on the futon in the tiny living room of our apartment in Baltimore, I felt wholly disconnected. I was too far away from home. Mom edited herself to keep me from worrying. I knew I wasn't getting all the information.

In a conversation with her earlier that week, I'd heard something new. A shift. She dropped her guard and hinted that Dad's mental state was changing. "There are these moments when I see him gazing off into the distance, and I feel like I can't reach him," she said, and I caught the waver in her voice. "When I regain his attention, it's like he doesn't know he wasn't with me the whole time." A sad weariness buried inside her final sentence.

After hanging up, I dialed Mark. I needed him to give me the real story. The unabridged version. He was in his third year of his pediatrics residency at the Izaak Walton Killam Hospital in Halifax. He and Ellen lived in a downtown apartment about fifteen minutes from my parents. He remained the inside track for those of us who lived away.

"Dad's pretty low," he said after some urging. He, too, straddled that line of trying not to worry me when there wasn't much I could do. "Mom's beyond exhausted."

"I'm coming home," I decided.

The private girls' school where I taught closed for Thanksgiving week, and Chris and I were already planning to drive from Baltimore to Nashua as soon as I finished teaching on Friday to spend the holiday with his parents and brother. I found a cheap, last-minute flight to Halifax from Boston. We drove the eight hours Friday night, and I flew out of Logan the next morning.

"Let's make it a surprise," I suggested to Mom when the logistics were set. "Don't tell Dad I'm coming." I did want to surprise him. More than that, though, I wanted the honest, authentic version of him. The one that wouldn't try to pretend that things were better than they were.

The customs agent stamped my passport, smiled for the first time, revealing deep dimples in his cheeks, and said, "Enjoy your visit."

"Thank you." I forced a smile in return. I stepped beyond his booth and moved to the side as he called the next passenger in line. The wall next to me displayed colorful, oversized canvases depicting Nova Scotia tourist attractions: bustling restaurants and shops on the Halifax Waterfront, military reenactors marching in formation on Citadel Hill, wooden lobster boats docked in the alcoves of quaint fishing villages on the South Shore, sea waves crashing against the giant rock ledge beneath the lighthouse at Peggy's Cove. Inviting images of the place I'd called home since the summer before I started college.

Just outside the frosted glass exit doors in front of me, I knew Mom was waiting. I tucked my passport into my schoolbag. I took extra time to put on my heavy winter coat and gather my things. On purpose, I slowed this part down. I slowed it down because I also knew that when I walked over that threshold and through those doors, a lot more would be waiting for me than just my mother.

—

Outside the bank of large rectangle windows lining the far length of the room, the steel sky threatened snow. The tall maples that reached up from the ravine behind the house had lost their leaves and between their naked branches was an uninhibited view of the Halifax Harbor in the distance. Choppy waves punctuated its surface; November snowstorms were not uncommon in Nova Scotia. Inside my parents' house, warmed by the gas stove in the corner and a cup of Earl Grey, I nestled at the end of the couch in the family room. I was reading *The Shipping News*. The book had sat on the white bedside table in my old bedroom when I'd arrived two days earlier, and last night, I started reading it. I already loved it. Quoyle and the rich cast of Newfoundlanders who inhabited the story felt like friends. Annie Proulx understood the ties to water and land that lived inside Maritimers. The ties that lived inside me.

Dad dozed beside me. His feet were propped up on my lap and his head rested against a throw pillow at the other end of the couch. His mouth was slightly open, and his breath exhaled in small wheezes. In the past two days, I'd gotten used to the drone of the small oxygen tank that traveled everywhere with him. A clear plastic tube coiled from the cylinder on the floor, hooked over his ears, and attached to two prongs in his nostrils. He'd pushed the prongs from his nose and they rested on his top lip. I decided not to try to readjust the tubes just now. He was still wearing his glasses. He looked peaceful, and I didn't want to disturb him. Mom was at the grocery store, and, for the moment, it was just the two of us.

My visit had consisted of variations on this same scene. With Mom on one side and me on the other, holding tightly to his elbows, we developed a system for steadying Dad on the stairs from the second to the main floor, so he could migrate from his bed to the couch. The journey from one locale to the other was enough to wear him out, and it would have been easier for me to just hang out with him in his bedroom, but he insisted on getting out of bed and coming downstairs to be with me. To sit back and listen as I described my students at Notre Dame Preparatory School, the prestigious Catholic girls' school where I taught. He wanted to hear me talk about my latest strategies for teaching them American and World History even though my college history minor made me less than an expert in either. He wanted to learn details of Chris's second year of graduate studies at the University of Maryland, to immerse himself in our world and picture the life we'd started away from here. In these moments, in this setting, I fell easily into my family role: ambassador of joy.

My arrival on Saturday was a genuine surprise. Before she left to pick me up from the airport under the guise of running some errands, Mom promised Dad she'd bring him back something special. I'm not sure what he expected, but he wasn't expecting me.

"I've got your present," Mom said with exaggerated cheer as she led me through the doorway into their bedroom. Dad rested on pillows propped against the pine headboard watching TV. He was dressed in faded sweats and his favorite blue polar fleece, which he called his "fuzzy." A cotton throw bunched around his feet. On our drive from the airport, Mom had tried to prepare me for the changes I'd see in him, using modifiers like "weaker" and "thinner." He was indeed thinner than when I'd seen him in August. His arms and legs looked lost in the bulk of his clothing. His cheekbones more pronounced. The shadowed skin around his eyes was slack.

But the word "weaker" was wrong. It did nothing to prepare me for the absolute frailty of his demeanor. Dad had always had this amazing presence as he moved through the world. He could fill a room with his confidence. A magnet attracting people without having to try. Now, he looked so small. I swallowed hard, but the lump lodged in my airway stayed put. The words came unbidden into my mind.

This is it.

Mark was sitting in the recliner beside the sliding glass patio door that led onto the small deck off of my parents' room. He stood up when Mom and I came in. I met his eyes and read his thoughts. *There was no way I could explain this over the phone.*

Dad turned his head at Mom's announcement about "the present." When he saw me, his face registered first confusion, then shock, and finally opened into the utter delight of recognition. "Melanie Joybells," he said in a hoarse whisper. He coughed and cleared his throat. "Where did you come from?"

"Hi, Daddy." I grinned and walked to the other side of the bed and climbed up beside him. I reached for his hand. Its warmth was reassuring. I kept my voice light. "I happened to be in the neighborhood, so I thought I'd stop by."

A sparkle flickered in his eyes, and his lips spread into a smile wide enough to expose the gap on the far-right side where his false tooth was supposed to be. A series of failed root canals a couple of years ago had led his dentist to pull the bicuspid and replace it with a fake one. The prosthetic never fit properly, and Dad was prone to remove it when it started pinching his gums, and then forget where he'd left it. Absurd locations where Mom found it became a running family joke. She'd discover it stashed away in the pockets of shirts or pants, wrapped in a napkin, or sitting at the bottom of empty water glasses. She'd opened a kitchen cabinet once and found the rogue tooth resting on the ledge. The previous summer, it had disappeared for good, and Dad hadn't bothered to replace it. I think it was a relief for him to be rid of it.

"I can't believe you're here. I'm so happy," he said. Just like that. No protests about the cost of the flight or the time away from Chris and our established plans or the inconvenience. No masking his weaknesses. No deflecting. Dad's "always make it look good" aura was gone and in its place, a rare and pure expression of what he was really feeling. With his hand still in mine, he shifted position and rested his head in my lap. I glanced at Mom, who sat on his other side. She was smiling, but tears gathered at the corners of her blue eyes. I pushed back against the threat of my own. I brushed the hair away from Dad's broad forehead. So soft and thin.

I didn't want to move. I didn't want to step beyond this moment into the moments that undoubtedly lay ahead. I traced the contours of his head with my hand, unable to take my eyes off of his face. This was still Dad. A yearning for something I could not name throbbed deep inside me. A need to protect him. To take care of him. To stop what was coming from coming.

I could not.

What I could do was give him the side of me he wanted. Needed. I could be the sunny daughter he adored. With a brightness I didn't quite feel dousing my words, I said, "You wouldn't believe the craziness at the airport in Boston! You have no idea how much Americans love their Thanksgiving."

Melanie Joybells had come home.

Now, I was content to sit at my end of the couch while Dad slept. I knew it comforted him to have me near. The pull was just as strong for me. I couldn't sit close enough. I couldn't touch him enough. I was the little girl me, clutching his pant leg or clinging to his neck to keep him that minute longer before he disappeared out the front door for a shift at the hospital or backed out of my bedroom after he'd tucked me in for bed. I was doing everything I could to keep from letting him go.

"Mel," Dad said. His voice startled me from the pages of my book. He was looking at me, his eyes intent behind his square glasses. "I need your help with something."

"Okay," I said before he explained what he wanted. Whatever it was, my answer would be the same. I would do anything for him.

"We need to do some 'elfing.'" He adjusted the oxygen prongs and straightened his glasses. At his movement, Abby sat up from where she'd been lying squeezed into the space between the couch and the coffee table. She rested her head on the cushion and nosed Dad's arm. He scratched behind her ears. Her tail thumped on the carpet. She, too, couldn't get close enough to him.

I folded the corner of the page and put down my book. "Elfing" was a longstanding tradition for us. He enlisted me to help him shop for Christmas, most often for my mother. When I lived at home, he and I would set aside one day during the holidays to browse in specialty jewelry stores for earrings or necklaces, or high-end women's boutiques for outfits she might like. He was never short on ideas, but he often needed me to consult or serve as his model for the gifts he was considering.

Christmas was Dad's specialty. He loved the music and the meaning. He particularly loved the presents. When it came to gifts, he was a go big or go home kind of guy, and he was all about the showstopper: the gift that would catch one (or all) of us by surprise. The year I was ten, my brothers and I followed a treasure hunt of rhyming clues all over town to discover we were going to Disney World. Our bags already packed. We flew out Christmas night.

In most avenues of his life, Dad avoided extravagance. It made him uncomfortable. In the post-World War II era, he'd watched his parents struggle to afford basics. An orange in his stocking was a luxury. That childhood struggle had fed his desire to make Christmas a magical time. He would figure out that one gift that would inevitably flood us with delight. We were never disappointed. Every year, he and Mom would set a spending limit, and every year he'd break it. When Dad disappeared for a few hours on Christmas Eve for "a little last-minute shopping," we knew something special was coming our way.

Christmas was five weeks away. Five uncertain weeks. Nobody was talking about those weeks. Talking about them would mean talking about whether Dad was going to be alive this Christmas.

But now, Dad pointed to a basket under the coffee table, piled high with magazines and said, "Grab me the L.L. Bean catalog." He wanted me to help him shop. To order gifts for Christmas. Five weeks away.

The lump in my throat was back.

The previous night, after Dad went to bed, Mom sat with me for a while at the kitchen table, sipping from a cup of decaf coffee, and told me again she was afraid pieces of his mind were slipping away.

"Most days, he's still himself, but there have been a few where he's barely talked at all," she said, balancing her mug in her hands. "And those days, his thoughts seem muddled, like he's struggling to put them together."

"Is dementia a complication of AIDS?" I couldn't imagine my dad's mind vanishing.

"It can be if there's some sort of infection impacting his brain."

Dad was no longer considered "under treatment." After the push to get to Mark and Ellen's wedding, he'd put a stop to everything. No new tests. No more experimental drugs. The only medical care he received was palliative. If something was going on in his brain, we had no real way of knowing.

"Lately, when we're sitting down here or lying in bed, he'll say my name," Mom said, standing up and carrying the cups from the table to the dishwasher. Her slippered feet padded across the floor. "But then, when I answer 'Yes,' he just stares at me and doesn't speak. It's like he's trying to tell me something, but he can't find the words."

I wished I could find the words now to determine whether Dad was thinking the same things I was thinking. Since I'd been home, he hadn't talked about being sick. About dying. It had never been the kind of talk we had. Selfishly, I wish now he would talk about it, if only for me. He'd always been the person who told me how to do things. And I didn't know how to do any of this. I was not ready. I wanted to tell him that I needed him to stay longer. That I needed him to still be here at Christmas, when Chris and I would be back home again. That anything else was unbearable.

Instead, I reached for the catalog, passed it to Dad, and asked, "Where should we start?"

"We need my credit card." His voice was energized.

He didn't know where his wallet was. I didn't ask him to remember where he put it the last time he'd left the house. I wasn't sure he remembered the last time he'd left the house. I lifted his legs off my lap and got up to hunt for it, hoping to find it somewhere in the large adjacent kitchen. It was not anywhere on the counter. I checked the shelves of the built-in desk next to the pantry cabinet. Luck was on my side. The wallet was there beside a set of car keys. I grabbed it, a pen, and the cordless telephone and returned to my spot. Dad propped his feet back in my lap.

"Mom needs new slippers," he said, leafing through the pages of the catalog. He scrutinized the images and his forehead creased in concentration. I knew he hadn't been able to read much lately. Headaches came on quickly and blurred his vision.

"Let me look," I said. He handed me the catalog. I flipped to the footwear section.

"She likes the kind that are like moccasins. Not the ones that only cover her toes and flap on her heels."

"How about these?" I held the catalog up so he could see the choices.

"I like the ones without the bow."

I took a pen and circled the item number. "Size nine and a half, right? What about color?"

"Blue," we both said at once. Blue was my mother's favorite color. When given a choice, she'd always choose blue. I often teased her about her wardrobe that was composed of different shades of the same color.

"Now sweaters," Dad said.

For the next half hour, we scoured the entire women's section of the catalog, circling a few more items for Mom along the way: a bathrobe, a sweater. It didn't take long for Dad's momentum to begin to wilt. He talked less and let me do most of the choosing.

"Should we take a break?" I asked when he put his head back and shut his eyes.

He didn't say anything, and I started to close the catalog. Then he began to wiggle his toes. His eyes opened, and he propped himself up on his elbows so he could see his feet. "Find these socks," he said, continuing with the toe action. "They are warm and don't itch. These are really cozy socks."

I took a closer look at the blue cotton socks covering his squirming feet and then looked back through the catalog. I found them. One hundred percent cotton ragg socks. $9.95. "Who are they for?" I asked.

"Get some in every color," he said.

"There are like ten different colors, Dad!" I pointed to the product description.

"Perfect. Order them all."

"All of them? Who are they for?" I asked again.

"Everybody," he said simply, and then added, "I think you all could use some warm and really cozy socks this Christmas."

Tears assembled just above my lower lashes. I didn't speak. If I did, I would cry. And if I started crying, I might never stop.

I didn't argue spending $100 on close to a dozen pairs of socks. When Dad got an idea in his head, there was no dissuading him. I picked up the phone and dialed the number for L.L. Bean. A friendly operator with a distinctive Maine accent took my order.

"How's the weathah up they-uh?" she asked after I read off the credit card numbers and gave her the shipping information.

"We might be getting some snow," I said, looking again at the darkening clouds out the windows. The wind had picked up, and the tree branches swayed about in a dance without rhythm.

"Thaht'll make things festive foah the holidays," she said. Her words nudged me back to the reality of what I was doing.

I glanced in Dad's direction. He was looking out the window. He'd gotten lost somewhere in his head while I'd been talking on the phone. A faraway expression glazed his eyes.

"I guess," I said to the operator, desperate now to end the call. I didn't want to be talking on the phone to a stranger in Maine about festive, snow-covered holidays. I didn't want to be ordering these presents. These presents I'd have to wrap in shiny paper and give out myself because Dad likely wouldn't be there to do it.

I set the phone down on the coffee table. Dad breathed in deeply. "There," he said and rested his head on the pillow. He closed his eyes. I circled my hands around his cozy-socked feet and sat like that, watching his chest rise and fall in a steady rhythm, until he fell asleep.

After All This Time, It's Time

Friday, December 8, 1995

THE LIGHTS WERE dim in the auditorium when I slipped into a row near the back and sat down next to my friend Maria, our Spanish teacher. Around us, students crowded the seats, high school girls dressed in the signature uniform of Notre Dame Preparatory School: bright blue dresses with white, Peter Pan collars and black and white saddle shoes. The colorful, grosgrain ribbons wrapped around their high ponytails were the only personalized accessories allowed. Their raucous chatter hushed as the first strums on the guitar echoed through the space and signaled the start of the weekly liturgy. I stood with everyone else and trained my eyes forward.

The bottom of the raised stage was draped with green garlands and red, velvet bows. A tall evergreen, its white lights twinkling behind the ornaments decorating its boughs, stood beside the small group of musicians—a few teachers and staff members—who led the familiar carols that opened the service before the formal beginning of the Mass. This prep school where I'd taught for a year and a half was one of the oldest Catholic girls' schools in the region, and its central roots of faith were on full display in these weekly school-wide worship gatherings. My Protestant upbringing did not expose me to the beauty of liturgical rituals: the formality of language, the sacred images and icons, the communal chants and prayers. I'd encountered something deeply moving in the repetitive practice of these community traditions.

I tried to relax into this late-morning break from the day's teaching and pushed thoughts of semester exam prep and papers waiting to be graded from my mind. I joined the singing on the chorus of "O Come, O Come Emmanuel." *Rejoice! Rejoice! Emmanuel shall come to thee, O Israel.* I'd sung these words my whole life and they rolled off my tongue with ease but hearing them fill the air and mingle with the soft guitar chords tugged at my unsteady composure.

Since my return from Halifax two weeks earlier, I'd been trying to keep it all together. Trying to ignore the realities of Dad's downward progression laid bare on that spur-of-the-moment trip home and trying to focus on doing my job. Teaching my classes. Breathing in and out.

Yet, in the stillness of night when I was practicing the breathing in and out, unable to manufacture sleep, I couldn't escape the images of Dad's frail and weakened body, so much frailer and weaker than when I'd seen him in August. I couldn't stop hearing his labored breathing and the persistent drone of his oxygen tank. I couldn't forget the child-like helplessness in his eyes. No matter how much I tried, I couldn't deny that he was teetering dangerously close to the unthinkable.

But there was no telling how long this teetering could last.

"It's a slow decline," the doctor said.

"He's holding steady," Mark said.

"Go back and finish out the semester. It's only four weeks until Christmas, and you'll be home again," Mom said.

So, despite the urgent voice inside me that said, "Stay," I listened to them. I didn't cry, and I even managed an upbeat smile when I hugged Dad goodbye, pushing back the thoughts that it was possibly the last time. I came back to Baltimore. To Chris. To our life and responsibilities. To this season of Advent. This season of waiting for what comes next.

Around me, the voices of seven hundred girls carried the sacred words and harmonies of hope. Hope I'd wrapped into my consciousness and clung to for ten years so I could stay standing. But in that instant, my hold loosened. It happened so quickly and unexpectedly. I felt myself let go. A certainty gripped my stomach and made me double over, rest my hands on my knees, pull air into my heaving lungs. I knew. I knew our hope was gone. Our waiting was over. Dad was going to die soon, and I was a thousand miles away.

The carols continued without pause, transitioning to, "O Little Town of Bethlehem." I straightened, conscious of drawing attention. Tears splashed onto my cheeks. Uncontrolled sobs rippled through me, swallowed by the music. Maria had observed my distress. Since returning from my Thanksgiving trip, I'd opened up to her a bit. She reached for my hand and clutched it in hers. She was crying too.

It was too much: the music, the words, the distance. Time was up, and this auditorium, this school, this city—this was not where I wanted to be. Was not where I needed to be.

"I have to go," I mouthed as I pushed my way past Maria to the aisle. With my head down, I staggered to the back of the auditorium and lurched through the heavy doors into the empty corridor. The joyful sounds of Christmas faded behind me. Even though I was alone, I felt exposed, my emotions too raw. These tears stored all of the other tears from all of the other moments that had led to this moment.

I believed they would never stop.

—

Later that afternoon I sat on the futon in the living room of our apartment, cradling the cordless phone in my hands, hesitating to make the call to Halifax, unsure about my own instincts. Outside the sliding glass doors, snowflakes scattered on the wind and speckled the patio railing. My coat, boots, bag, and books were strewn across the carpeted floor where I'd shed them when I'd stumbled through the door a few minutes earlier.

My breakdown and retreat from liturgy had not gone unnoticed. Moments after I'd clicked the lock on the door of the faculty bathroom next to the Social Studies office and collapsed on the closed toilet seat, my face buried in my hands, my sobs muffled by my fingers, a soft knock startled me.

"Mel? Can you let me in?"

I stood, and with trembling hands, turned the metal knob and opened the door to Kathleen, a fellow Social Studies teacher and dear friend. Her face reflected concern and intimate understanding. Two years earlier, she'd lost her father to cancer. This connection had made her someone I could confide in over the last few months. She was only three years older than I was, so despite how guarded I'd been with my situation, she understood this was all happening too soon.

"What's going on?" she asked as she pulled me into a tight hug. Despite her small frame, her support felt huge.

"I don't know," I managed to gasp, wiping my eyes and nose with the wad of toilet paper I clutched in my fist. "The season, the music … I just have a feeling that …" I couldn't complete the sentence.

"Go home," she said, guiding me into the adjacent office. "I'll cover your afternoon classes," she added before I could protest. She helped me get my things together. "Go home," she said again, her voice firmer. She was urging me to do more than take the afternoon off.

I was so grateful as I hugged her one more time. Grateful for her comfort in that moment, and grateful for the comfort I knew she'd have waiting for me when I returned on the other side of this. Whatever this turned out to be.

Now, wrapping a throw blanket around my shoulders, I curled against a pillow and tucked my feet underneath me. I stared out the window at the swirling snowflakes, trying to settle my thoughts before pressing the numbers on the phone. I wanted to talk to Mom. I wanted her to validate this feeling that had dropped into my gut during liturgy, this feeling that something was happening. I wanted to beg her to tell me exactly what that something was. And, most of all, I wanted her to tell me to come home.

I hesitated, though, my fingers poised over the dial. As long as I didn't call, what I was feeling was just a feeling, and feelings could be wrong.

I looked at the potted Norfolk pine in the corner. Last year, celebrating our first Christmas together, Chris and I had strung it with white lights and decorated it with heavy ornaments that bent the thin branches. This year, it remained bare.

The phone jangled in my hand, and I jumped.

I pushed the talk button, and answered with a faltering, "Hello?"

"Melanie? It's Sister Helen."

My headmistress. The stately, no-nonsense nun whose quiet nature did not diminish the largeness of her presence. She'd been at the school's helm for twenty-five years, but she'd been a beloved part of the academic community for close to sixty. My only other direct experience with Catholic nuns was when I was eleven and studied piano lessons at a music school in Moncton, New Brunswick, administered by the sisters of Notre-Dame-du-Sacre-Coeur. That venture ended abruptly on the day I came out of my lesson and showed Mom my bruised knuckles from the sister rapping my hands with a ruler every time I stumbled over a note. I'd never had to go back. So, despite Sister Helen's kind demeanor, I'd always been a little frightened of her.

I straightened my back and said, "Sister, I'm sorry I didn't tell you I was leaving school ..."

She interrupted and her tone was sympathetic. "Melanie, I think you should take some time. I think you should go be with your family. With your father." I hadn't talked to Sister Helen about my situation at home because, until today, it hadn't impacted my ability to do my work. In the small community of our school, word traveled fast. My guess was that Kathleen had spoken to her. I was grateful I didn't have to repeat the story.

"I'm not sure it's time, sister," I said. Stacks of ungraded quizzes and papers remained on my shelf in the Social Studies office. Two chapters in the thick history text remained to be covered to get my sophomores through the end of the Constitutional Convention before the exam in January. "I don't want to leave the girls hanging. I think I'll be able to finish out the semester." There was one full week of school left and then two days the following week before Christmas vacation. What if I used up all of my personal days now if I didn't need to? What would happen when I did need to?

"Melanie," Sister Helen said, her voice unwavering. "I want you to understand what I'm saying. Your job will be here. Your students will be here. We will be here. I'm telling you to take all the time you need. However much time that is. Everything will still be here when you get back."

I couldn't speak right away. I was so used to dealing with things on my own that when confronted with genuine care I didn't know how to respond. I squeezed my burning eyes shut and clenched my teeth, willing the remnants of my earlier sobs to stay put. There was so much I wanted to say, but I couldn't find the right words.

"Thank you, sister," I finally exhaled.

"Think about it. Let me know when you decide so we can get your classes covered." She paused, then added, "This time is sacred, Melanie. Do whatever you need to do."

I wished someone could tell me what that was.

"I will, sister. I, I'm just so ... Thank you."

"We will all remember you in our prayers." She hung up.

I pushed the "off" button and let the phone rest on my palm for only an instant before I dialed the 902 area code for Nova Scotia and pressed the other numbers.

Holding the phone against my ear with one hand, I clasped the fringed edge of the blanket to my neck with the other.

After two rings, a bubbly voice answered, "Hello?"

I wasn't expecting Aunt Gloria, my dad's sister, to pick up. I'd forgotten that she was there. She'd been in Halifax for the last week, visiting from her home in Columbus, Ohio, giving my mom some respite, spending time with Dad. I was in no state to talk to her, but I tried to make my voice sound normal when I said, "Oh, hi, Aunt Gloria. It's Melanie. Is my mom there?"

"She's out getting her hair cut. I told her she just had to go even though she wasn't going to. Your dad and I have been having a great old time watching the container ships coming into the harbor and chatting about all sorts of things. He's been awake quite a bit today, all comfy, sitting right up against his pillows. A little bit foggy, but alert. Let me put him on the phone; I'm sure he'd love to talk to you." All of this came out on one extended breath in a chipper tone that I could tell was for Dad's benefit, not mine. I had no time to interrupt, no time to say that I'd rather wait to talk to Mom when she got home, that I wasn't composed enough to talk to Dad.

Instead, I heard some muffled conversation as the phone shifted hands, and then, "Hel-lo?" Dad's voice was groggy and slow to pronounce each syllable, a pause for breath in between.

My eyes filled with all the tears of the day, and I struggled to speak. I'd called home almost every evening since Thanksgiving, and often, after she'd given me the standard update, "No big changes," Mom would give Dad the other extension so he could listen to our conversation. He didn't say much, the work of putting logical sentences together too tiring for him these days. Now, though, it was just the two of us again.

"Hi, Daddy," I said.

"Meligans," he said, again punctuating each syllable with an intake of air. "What are you doing?"

I watched the clouds drifting through the sky. Gray on gray. I doubted Dad knew what day it was or what time it was. Doubted he knew that I was calling in the middle of a Friday when I was supposed to be teaching.

"I came home a little early from school."

"Sick?"

"No, not sick. I was feeling a little sad." This was like a conversation I might have with a child. Paring things down to the simplest of statements.

"Well," he said, and then, for a long minute, he didn't say anything. I listened to his shallow breaths, worrying that I'd confused him and triggered something in his mind that he couldn't quite form into meaning.

"I'm okay, Dad," I tried to reassure, regretting that I'd said anything.

"Well," he said again. And then, with a sudden liveliness to his voice, "We'll be down there soon. Soon. When we get down there, it'll be all right."

He'd gone somewhere away from our conversation. Somewhere away from the reality of what was going on. Somewhere in his memory or somewhere in an alternate world where life was moving forward, plans were being made. Somewhere that had him, and Mom, I guessed, traveling south to see me.

I rested my head on the cushion. My tears soaked into the fabric and left a wet spot under my cheek. This was how it was going to feel. This empty space that was opening between us—it was going to feel like being in this void all the time.

"Dad, I'm going to call back in a little while when Mom is home. We can talk some more then, okay?"

There was no response, and from the steady rhythm of his breathing, I assumed he'd fallen asleep. I wondered if Aunt Gloria had stayed in the room or whether she'd left him alone for these few minutes.

Then, "Love you." The two words slurred together, almost indecipherable, but I heard them. I hauled myself out of the emptiness. He was still here. For right now, he was still here.

"I love you, Dad. I'll see you soon," I whispered and hung up the phone.

Calm Before

Saturday

BEFORE I TURNED to board my flight at the gate of Baltimore-Washington International Airport, I clung to Chris for a long time. My arms wrapped around his solid frame, and my body drew on his strength. Strength that was propping us both up. He was not coming with me and detaching from him felt like leaving a crucial piece of myself behind. He had two more classes at the University of Maryland to get through on Monday and Tuesday. A paper to finish, and a final exam. Last night, as we'd rushed to coordinate my exit: booking the flight, packing, making the necessary calls to extract me from all of my responsibilities in the coming days, we'd decided he should wait.

When I got there, I'd know better whether it was time for him to fly in.

Ever practical, Mom had almost talked me out of going when I'd finally spoken to her yesterday. She'd fretted about me missing school. She didn't feel like there was anything I could do by coming home right now. "I'm going to need you *after*," she'd said, the load of the sentence falling on that one preposition. "When this is all over, that's when I'm going to need you the most."

I wanted to tell her that this was about me. About what I needed. About this unnamed feeling that forecast my deepest fears. But I didn't. How could I?

I agreed to wait for a day or two before making plans. But as soon as I hung up the phone with her, I dialed Mark. "Should I come home?"

I asked, not bothering to disguise the messiness of my distress. "Is it time?" To ask this question out loud, this question I never asked, was wrenching.

He hesitated. Mark was not an alarmist, and I knew he'd avoid painting too dire a picture if he wasn't sure. But he didn't answer my question. Instead, he asked one of his own. The one I'd needed somebody to ask. "Do you want to come home, Mel?"

"Yes."

"Let me talk to Mom."

Relief washed over me. Because I still straddled that middle place between my role as child and my role as adult, I felt like I needed Mom's permission.

Less than twenty minutes later, she called back. "If you think you can sort things out there, then maybe you should come home," she said.

I boarded the plane and found my seat. This first leg to Philadelphia was a weekday commuter route, but apparently not a Saturday afternoon favorite. No one sat next to me.

The plane taxied, and I leaned my head against the window and watched the tarmac blur into a smoky cloud. I closed my eyes as the flight attendant began her passenger safety demonstration and indicated the emergency exits at the front, rear, and sides of the aircraft. The plane lifted off the ground and the drone of her voice mingled with the roar of the engines and lulled me toward sleep. I surrendered to its pull.

The Music Fades

Sunday

I SAT AT the end of Mom and Dad's queen-sized bed, a pillow positioned between my back and one of the pine posts that attached to the footboard. I'd been there before. The scene mirrored the ones from August, when Dad was so sick before Mark and Ellen's wedding. The humming oxygen machine on the floor. The metal IV pole with dripping meds next to the bed. Dad, his shrunken form buried beneath the heavy comforter, coasting on a morphine-induced sleep, brief interludes of alertness interrupting now and then.

August, I realized, had been the rehearsal for now.

The skeletal angles of Dad's face, the permanent lines of tension in his forehead, the sunken hollows in his cheeks and around his eyes, the ashy hue of his skin—these things told me the real show had begun.

I'd arrived the night before without any fuss. It was late when Mark picked me up at the airport. He loaded my suitcase into the trunk of his car, turned to me, and said the words, "Here we go." I felt their meaning. Mark and Ellen had been camping out at our parents' for the last few nights, Mark's medical training the gift that let Dad be at home.

Though the house on Julie's Walk was dark when we pulled into the driveway, Mom, dressed in her blue housecoat tied loosely over her nightgown, was waiting up to see me. Dark circles lined her tired eyes. "I'm so glad you're home," she said, hugging me against her too-thin frame. The last few weeks had been especially hard on her, worrying and caretaking had wreaked equal havoc on her ability to sleep or eat.

"Me too," I said.

We didn't linger over conversation. We were all exhausted. I climbed the carpeted stairs toward the guestroom and stood for a minute in the darkened hallway outside Mom and Dad's bedroom. I listened for a long time to the sound of Dad's breathing, soothed by its steady rhythm.

This morning, a mix of wet snow and rain fell outside, and low, murky clouds cloaked the normally expansive view of the harbor from my parents' bedroom. Awake and in a semi-upright position, Dad sank into a collection of puffy pillows that bolstered him from all sides, his body too weak to support itself.

He hadn't said more than a few words since I'd settled into my spot on the bed, but from the light of awareness in his eyes I could tell he knew me. I was not sure that his mind, muddled by the dripping medication whose only job now was to keep him comfortable and pain-free, registered that I'd arrived from somewhere away, that I hadn't been with him all along. It didn't matter. I was here, and so was he.

Mom and Aunt Gloria sat in chairs pulled close to the bed. Dad listened to our chatter. Aunt Gloria, a fountain of conversation in any circumstance, tossed questions my way.

"Do you like living in Baltimore, Melanie?"

"How's your teaching?"

"What's Chris working on these days?"

"Did I tell you that Julie's considering joining the Peace Corps?"

I answered each one and tried to quell the twinges of resentment I felt at her presence and polite dialogue about things that didn't matter to me right now. I loved her. I was so grateful for the help she'd been giving Mom over the past week. But sharing this most intimate and vulnerable of times with anyone outside our immediate family circle, anyone who hadn't traveled this rutted road of illness and secrecy and isolation and despair at close range, felt oddly uncomfortable.

Ellen walked into the room and Mark followed, a purple Popsicle in his hand. The kitchen freezer was stocked with Popsicles, among the only things that Dad would still eat. Dad turned his head at the shuffle of their footsteps and his face broke into a huge smile. "You came all the way up here to give me a Pop—" he exclaimed at the same instant Mark bit the top off the frozen treat. Dad's mouth turned into the crestfallen pout of a little boy who had just had a toy snatched away. Mark froze, the Popsicle suspended in midair. Guilt wrote into his expression, and with his words garbled by the chunk of ice on his tongue, he said weakly, "You want the rest?"

A giggle escaped my lips. Mark's primary focus in the last days and weeks had been anticipating and meeting all of Dad's physical needs. The inflated look of disappointment that hijacked Dad's face over this apparent infraction struck me as ironic. And funny. So I laughed. We all did. Even Dad joined in the levity, a smile replacing the pout, though I'm not sure he understood the joke. I wiped tears and welcomed the chance to release them this way.

"Dad, when I saw your face …" I said, still laughing as Mark disappeared out the door to retrieve another Popsicle from the freezer.

The moment was fleeting. Dad turned his head on the pillow and closed his eyes. Mark returned, but the Popsicle was off the radar now. Fatigue had slipped in, and it was pulling Dad away.

Mom reached for the remote on the bedside table, pointed it at the TV on the low stand against the wall, and pushed the ON button. "How about some church?" she said and flipped the channel to the broadcast of a large congregation seated in wooden pews, their heads bowed as the voice of the minister finished a prayer. Dad opened his eyes and focused for a minute on the screen.

My dad had never been a fan of televangelists, but he'd always enjoyed watching Robert Schuller's *Hour of Power* screened from inside the massive Crystal Cathedral in Garden Grove, California. Dad loved the music—the traditional hymn-based repertoire performed by a stellar choir and full orchestra. Famed pianist, Roger Williams, was often a guest accompanist and performer in these Sunday morning services.

Hundreds of red-leafed poinsettias decorated the raised platform at the front of the cathedral sanctuary, and the congregation joined the choir and orchestra to sing "O Come All Ye Faithful." I wanted to block out these reminders that time was ticking forward and Christmas was stealing closer.

The carols pacified Dad, though. He closed his eyes again. His face relaxed and his mouth settled into a half-smile. It was hard to know if he was awake or sleeping.

A soloist stepped onto the cathedral platform and began a beloved hymn, "It is Well with My Soul." She sang the opening words in a clear soprano voice. "When peace, like a river, attendeth my way / When sorrows like sea billows roll."

I was ten the summer week I spent at Word of Life, a Christian camp nestled in the Adirondack Mountains. It was my first sleep-away camp experience, and I'd loved it. At the end of each day, before trailing back to our cabins behind the bobbing beams of our flashlights, we all gathered in the mess hall for a time of singing and prayer with the camp's director. One evening, his wife stood up to sing, but first, she told us a story.

At the end of the 1800s, a rich Chicago lawyer named Horatio Spafford planned a holiday for his family. While he stayed in Chicago to wrap up some business, he sent his wife and four daughters ahead on an England-bound ship. The ship sank midway across the Atlantic and though his wife survived the tragedy, all of his daughters drowned. Spafford set sail to reunite with his grieving wife in England. When his ship crossed the area where his daughters had drowned, he penned the words to the hymn, "It is Well with My Soul."

"Can you imagine the pain he must have felt in that moment?" The director's wife had asked, her eyes shining with tears. "But in his deepest grief, this man relied on his faith. He turned to God for comfort and was able to find it." The music started, and she sang the hymn. I'd probably heard it before, but this time, enthralled by its history, I listened closely to the words. "Whatever my lot, Thou hast taught me to say / It is well, it is well, with my soul."

The hymn had since been my favorite. And it had long been one of Dad's favorites too. When he sat at the piano and folded one piece of music into another, his fingers seemingly choosing at random, "It is Well with My Soul" inevitably found its way into the set.

The soloist's voice resonated from the TV into the hush of the bedroom. "And Lord, haste the day, when the faith shall be sight / The clouds be rolled back as a scroll." Dad stirred on the bed. In one slow motion, he lifted his head off the pillow and leaned his body forward so he was sitting upright. He stretched his arms out and held them in front of him for a beat. And then, in a smooth cadence to the continuing notes of the music, his hands carved the air. Up and down, side to side, he gracefully followed the tempo and rhythm of the hymn through the gradual crescendo of the final verse. "The trump shall resound, and the Lord shall descend / Even so, it is well with my soul."

The rest of us watched, transfixed by his movements, this unexpected energy. An image from my childhood drifted near: me with my legs dangling above the floor, pressed against Dad on the piano bench, mesmerized by the magic in those hands that could produce the beautiful melodies simply by pressing down on the white and black keys. That same awe settled on my skin as Dad conducted the hymn's last triumphant bars.

A fierce longing swelled inside me. I wanted everything to stop. To freeze right here, right now with "It is Well with My Soul."

But the music died out. Dad's arms dropped to his sides, and he leaned back onto his mountain of pillows, eyes closed. He was asleep in seconds. His breaths were wheezy, but constant. I pushed my outstretched leg against his foot, feeling through the blanket its shape against my calf. The gulf I felt opening between us stretched wider each time he went. The ache that stayed behind was the thing I couldn't bear.

On His Way
Monday

DAD WAS LEAVING.

On Sunday night, while Ellen and I drove the fifteen minutes to King Wah Restaurant on Quinpool Road to pick up Chinese take-out for everyone, he'd decided to start heading out. When we walked into the kitchen with the stapled paper bags holding various entrees, Mom and Mark met us with the news that something had shifted in the thirty minutes we'd been gone. Dad had stopped responding. The consciousness that had been there earlier in the day had disappeared.

"I need you," I said to Chris when I called him later that night. "I need you here. Dad is dying." I'd been repeating those words to myself since Friday but hearing them aloud made my whole body go cold.

"I know, Mel. I'm trying to get there," Chris said. With all the Christmas travel, flights were heavily booked. He'd gotten a seat on one arriving on Tuesday. I was terrified he'd be too late.

"I don't think I can do this part without you," I whispered into the phone.

"I'll be there soon," he promised before hanging up.

Having missed the actual moment when Dad began his departure, all I could do was sit beside his bed and cling to what was left, not at all certain what that was.

He lay on his back. Supported by two pillows, his head tilted to the side. His eyes were half open, glassy, and vacant. His legs and arms jerked sporadically, and sometimes his face contorted, his forehead creasing and his eyes squeezing shut. Most of the time, though, he was so, so still.

His breathing had changed. The steady rhythm had been replaced by an irregular pattern of short, shallow pants in rapid succession followed by widening gaps with no breaths at all.

"It's time to come," Mom had told my other brothers, Michael and David, who were halfway across the country, both immersed in writing exams—David, his first college finals at Queen's University in Kingston, Ontario, and Michael, midterms for his first semester of law school at the University of Toronto. Now, after dropping everything and boarding last minute flights, they were somewhere in the air, reaching toward home.

At the same time, Aunt Gloria was on a plane back to Columbus to the support of her husband, my Uncle Stanley, and her long-time friends, and to the welcome comfort of her own home. With nothing but appreciation for the time she'd spent here, Mom had urged her to go. For Gloria's sake. For our sake. This part we had to do alone, but "we" all had to get here.

It was sometime Monday afternoon, but I was losing track of the hours. Mark and Ellen had been making the airport runs. I'd encouraged Mom to go lie down for a little while. Though Mark and I checked in sporadically and tried to get her to take a break, she'd sat up most of the night. Now, fighting a migraine, she could barely stay upright. I hoped she'd sleep.

Snow flurries persisted, but nothing accumulated. Long icicles hung from the edge of the roof, and the sky wore this dull grayness indefinitely. Soft saxophone played the lilting notes of "Away in a Manger," the five-disc CD player in the corner alternating between different Christmas albums. Kenny G's *Miracles: The Holiday Album* seemed to win the random shuffle more often than the rest of the CDs.

I reached for Dad's hand and squeezed. There was no answering grip. His fingers curled, and I extended each one so I could lace my own fingers in between. Dad's jaw was slack, his mouth open. With my other hand, I traced his lips with ice to keep them from chapping.

Fuck you, Kenny G! I screamed in my head as another of his album's songs, "Have Yourself a Merry Little Christmas," invaded the space. I hoped the music comforted Dad, but in these instances when Christmas's cues knocked against death's presence, my frayed nerves caught fire, and I had to fight the impulse to pick up the bowl of ice from the nightstand and chuck it at the sound system, silencing the saxophone for good.

I shifted my focus back to the unbearable rendering of my father on the bed. A pair of wishes dueled inside of me. *Don't let him know he's like this. Let him still be there somewhere.* I couldn't release either one.

"Everyone's coming, Dad," I said, leaning close to his ear. I didn't know if he could hear me, but I talked anyway. "David and Michael and Yvonne and Chris. They'll be here soon. Just hold on, okay?" I was asking a lot, but I couldn't help it. I was not ready. So much time stretched behind us. All those years of waiting. But now, as I felt the present moment rushing forward, I understood that none of it could ever have been enough.

Counting Silence
Tuesday

SIXTY-THREE. THAT was the record amount of space in between Dad's breaths. Sixty-three agonizing seconds.

"It's called Cheyne-Stokes," Mark had explained yesterday when the pattern of Dad's breathing took on this rhythmic sequence of accelerating and deepening breaths that then slowed and diminished to no breathing at all for a period before starting all over again. "It's another sign that his body is shutting down."

I'd been counting the silence all day. I held my own breath while I stared at Dad's motionless chest, waiting for the cycle to restart. And it did. Even after one interval that stretched to an impossible sixty-three seconds, Dad gasped a quick succession of breaths, and I slowly exhaled the air from my lungs.

Time slowed with Dad's breathing. Maybe it was because Dad's breathing had become our central focus. Everything else seemed like another place. Somewhere I used to live.

Chris reclined in a chair at the end of the bed, his legs stretched out, his feet propped on the footboard. He dozed off and on. When I'd picked him up at the airport earlier that evening, I'd hugged him tightly, letting my tears fall unchecked. I didn't have to try to find words anymore for what was happening. He could see for himself. There was a comforting certainty in his presence. A necessary glimpse of a future beyond now. Beyond these seconds between Dad's breaths.

Everybody had made it home: Michael and David, Michael's wife, Yvonne. Chris was the last to arrive. We navigated these hours of waiting in quiet solidarity. We were together, but separate, too, each of us lost in our own grief, our own anticipation of this loss. We sat at the bedside or down in the kitchen. We picked at the food that people from church had dropped off. We told stories. "Remember the time that ..." somebody would begin, and we'd laugh as the memories took shape. And then we'd cry because we understood that these stories, this history, were it. We'd always be reaching back from here to find Dad.

Mark was in charge. He took Dad's pulse. Monitored his respirations. Checked the mottling of his legs and arms that indicated their level of circulation. He adjusted the morphine drip when Dad seemed restless. We trusted him to limit Dad's pain. We looked to him to map this dying process for us. To tell us what we needed to know to survive it. He tried, but his knowledge had its borders.

Mom needed rest. We'd also been trying to take care of her. Mark gave her something to sleep, and the rest of us agreed to take two-hour shifts sitting with Dad through the night. "Promise you'll wake me up to take a shift too," Mom said, clutching my arm when I guided her into David's room to sleep on his bed while he took the couch downstairs. She'd been so strong. So selfless in how she cared for Dad. But she was crumbling in these final stages. In the faint light of the room, her face was pale, her eyes empty and lost.

"We will, Mom," I lied. We wouldn't wake her unless we had to.

It was our shift. Chris's and mine. The green numbers on the clock radio on the bedside table read a few minutes before midnight. At one o'clock, we'd wake Mark and Ellen to take our place, and we'd try to sleep.

The lamp on Mom's side of the bed was the one light on in the room. It bathed the space around the bed in a soft duskiness. Mom's long maple dresser against the wall and Dad's tall matching armoire in the far corner sank into the spaces the light couldn't reach. I stretched out next to Dad, lying semi-upright on my side, my face close to his. I rested my hand on his arm, comforted by the heat of his skin.

I talked to him, believing that somewhere inside this failing body, he was there, listening. I'd amended the message from yesterday, the one that pleaded with him to hold on. "You can go, Dad," I whispered as another cycle of respirations began. His weak chest muscles labored to pull these gasps of air into his lungs. It hurt me to watch. "You can stop." I cried as I voiced these words, tears salting my lips. "We'll all be okay." I didn't know if this was true. I didn't know if I'd ever be okay again. But Dad was so, so tired. This fight had been too long and too hard. We were all so tired.

I turned to look at Chris and saw that he was awake, his eyes concerned as he watched me. I wanted him to feel what I was feeling. To understand everything that gathered inside me. All this hurt of losing Dad. Of willing myself to let him go. But he hadn't loved him like I had. There hadn't been enough time. "I don't want to do this," I said, my voice cracking. "I really don't want to do this."

Chris dropped his legs down from the bed and leaned his body forward to press his hand against my leg. "I know," he said. "I know you don't."

We'd celebrated our first wedding anniversary at the end of July. Our life together, Chris's and mine, was barely started, and it had been marred by the downward progression of Dad's illness the whole time. And now we were facing this loss that had always hung near, tugging me toward home, threatening to snuff out all joy. He'd been so even and supportive. But sometimes I wondered if it was too much.

He seemed to sense where my thoughts had taken me. He pressed my leg again. "I'm here, Mel," he said, and there was no waver in his voice. "I'm here with you."

Set Adrift
Wednesday

"I CAN'T BELIEVE you let me sleep all night!" Mom exclaimed from her chair next to the bed when I stumbled into her bedroom, rumpled and rubbing my eyes. She held Dad's hand in both of hers. She looked better. She'd taken a shower and there was color in her cheeks. Her expression showed no signs of the exhausted confusion from the night before.

"When did you wake up?" I asked, glad she'd gotten good rest overnight.

"Only a little while ago. I really can't believe I slept all night." Despite her attempts at protest, I could tell she was grateful.

This morning, for the first time since I'd flown home on Saturday, the sun rose in a cloudless sky over the Halifax Harbor. It shone through the window, lighting the room and making everything seem sharper. An added curtain of warmth. Sea smoke misted over the distant water. Fluffy snow had collected overnight on the rooftops in the subdivision below our perch on Hemlock Ravine. The snow dusted the trees that stretched up behind the house and powdered the balcony railing.

After Mark and Ellen had taken over in the night, Chris and I slept for a few hours, curled together on the double bed in the guestroom next door. It was a restless sleep that had me wandering somewhere between awareness and unconsciousness. I sensed movement and sound but blended those things into the haze of fuzzy dreams. I woke early to slanting rays of light stealing in through gaps in the window blind, and I smiled into the heat I could feel on my face. For just a few seconds everything was peaceful. But then my eyes collected the details of the room: the soft pink walls, the paneled closet door, the suitcase overflowing with clothes in the far corner. I heard voices in the hallway. My mind rebooted, my smile disappeared, and I remembered.

We were back to waiting in these early morning hours, watching Dad hover on this precipice of dying. The labor of his breathing persisted, and the intervals still stretched between his gasps for air. We shuffled positions around the bed, but most of the time, I lay beside him, needing to be as close as I could. Sometimes we talked to each other, sometimes to Dad. Every few minutes, I leaned in, my lips close to his ear, my face brushing against the stubble on his cheek and whispered, "I love you, Dad. I love you so much." I'd used up all the other words, so I said this again and again.

"We need coffee," my brother Mike declared a little before nine o'clock. No one had thought to make a pot this morning. Too big an effort. There was a Tim Horton's just around the corner from the house—an easy drive.

"Donuts too," I said because I didn't drink coffee, and despite everything, I was hungry for something sweet.

He headed out the door. Mark and Ellen followed him to grab something down in the kitchen and David decided he'd take a quick shower. Chris sat in a recliner against the far wall, his head resting against the cushioned back.

I turned to Dad. His thin hair was disheveled, matted in spots and standing on end in others. It hadn't been combed or washed since Sunday, the last time he had sat up, the last time he was really with us.

"Mom," I said. "Would it be okay if I washed Dad's hair?"

"Yes," she said, looking at Dad as though she was noticing his appearance for the first time. "Good idea."

We went into their large en-suite bathroom, and Mom grabbed two towels and facecloths from the wicker basket sitting on the edge of the deep tub. She reached into the stand-up shower for a bottle of shampoo. I filled a plastic bowl with warm water.

I set the bowl down on the bedside table and dipped the facecloth into the water. Mom did the same with the second facecloth, deciding to wash Dad's feet and lower legs. Yvonne stood next to her at the bottom of the bed and held the towel. I wiped Dad's face and gently ran the damp cloth over his hair. I lifted his head off the pillow to wet the back, supporting his neck with one hand while I smoothed the facecloth over the curve of his skull with the other.

Dad changed color. In one quick rush, all pigment faded from his face and a ghostly gray mask took its place. It happened suddenly and definitively, and my stomach lurched because I knew what it meant.

"Mom," I said, my alarm shaping her name into a cry.

She looked up and gasped when she saw the color of Dad's face. "Oh, Melanie," she said, and tears filled her eyes. "Go get Mark."

Time sped and urgency thickened the air. I dropped the facecloth and rested Dad's head back on the pillow before flying out of the room to call for Mark down the staircase. He ran up, Ellen close behind. He looked at Dad. He pressed two fingers to Dad's neck to check his pulse. There was a new, coarse sound to Dad's rasping breaths now.

We called for David, and he rushed in, his hair dripping from the shower.

"It's happening," Mark said to us, his voice breaking, but these words weren't necessary.

"What about Michael?" I cried. He was still on the coffee run to Tim's. I grabbed the cordless phone from the dresser and dialed his cell phone. It rang over and over, but he didn't answer. I pushed down on my rising panic. He couldn't miss this moment. He had to be here. We all had to be here.

I dialed the number again.

"Hello?" his voice was hassled.

"Mike, you need to come right now," I said.

"I'm just in line, I'll be there soon," he said.

"You have to come now," I repeated. "It's time."

"I still have to pay for the coffee!" he said, irritation pressing on the words, and I knew by the absurdity of the statement he was not registering what I was saying.

"Just come," I pleaded and hung up the phone. I was crying. I returned to my spot beside Dad on the bed and reached for his hand, clutching it in mine. Chris stood and moved in close to me. I felt the pressure of his hand on my back.

With steady and knowing movements, Mark added more morphine to Dad's IV drip, enough to ease the labor of Dad's breathing. Of my three brothers, Mark looked the most like Dad. He had the same slope to his shoulders. The same subtle precision to his actions. He turned away from the IV pole and sat on the edge of the bed beside Mom. Ellen stood next to him and took his hand in hers. Tears streaked his cheeks. There was no more doctoring to do. Now, he could just be the son.

I was overcome with relief when I heard footsteps on the stairs, and Michael walked through the door, a question plastering his features. In one glance he swept our faces and then the bed, and he understood. His face softened, and he swallowed hard. He stood at the end of the bed with Yvonne and Dave and rested his hand on Dad's leg.

Dad's breaths were weaker and shallower. We pressed in, all of us reaching for a piece of him in these last minutes.

"Let's sing," Mom said, not wiping the tears that fell off her chin.

For a moment, we were quiet, and then Michael started, his baritone leading us into the first few bars of "How Great Thou Art." Faltering on the notes at first, the rest of us joined him, and we sang one familiar hymn after another: "Amazing Grace," "Great is Thy Faithfulness," "It is Well with My Soul." Their words came easily. Our voices blended into the natural harmonies cultivated from years of singing together as a family with Dad at the piano. We were all in, and I tried so hard to fasten to the hope echoed in the hymns, the hope that there was something beyond this death for Dad. It was fitting that the gospel music Dad played throughout our lives became the soundtrack for his death.

Michael picked up the worn Bible on the bedside table. His voice was steady as he read from the book of Psalms. "The Lord is my shepherd: I shall not want. He maketh me to lie down in green pastures; he leadeth me beside the still waters. He restoreth my soul." Outside, wind-swept snowflakes floated off the roof, their edges catching the light of the sun. "Yea, though I walk through the valley of the shadow of death, I will fear no evil, for thou art with me."

We watched Dad's sunken chest rise and fall. Rise and fall.

Then it stopped.

I knew he was gone. I felt him go at the same time that something inside of me ruptured. A low moan escaped my lips, and I buried my face against his shoulder. The rest of the world drifted into the distance. Muffled sobs and quiet words faded. I was the only one here, lying on the bed where a part of me would stay forever, clinging to Dad's still-warm hand.

Contradictions
Thursday

THE DAY AFTER Dad died, my brothers, sisters-in-law, Chris, and I convinced my mother that Dad would want her to have a new outfit for his funeral. So, we took her shopping. When we stepped through the glass-doored entrance to the Park Lane Mall on Spring Garden Road in Halifax, a blast of heat from the vents overhead hit us as we crossed the threshold—a sharp contrast to the frigid air that had numbed my face and fingers on the short walk from the car. I rubbed my hands together and glanced around. Even though it was December 14th, I startled at the merry scene that greeted me. While we'd inhabited the island of vigil at Dad's deathbed, Christmas had fully descended on the mainland.

Festive garlands that showcased giant ornaments with flickering white lights hung from the third-story ceiling. Red ribbons wrapped around posts, and potted poinsettias lined the walkways. An ornate evergreen, its branches adorned with tinsel and sparkling decorations, reached from the bottom floor to almost touch the glassed-in roof. Christmas carols serenaded the throng of holiday customers carrying oversized shopping bags, as they rode up and down the escalators and moved in a steady stream along the corridors between stores.

I felt wobbly and reached for Mom's hand. She clasped my fingers and stepped closer, and we leaned on each other for balance. The world felt out of focus, like I was seeing it through frosted glass. I couldn't reconcile all of this bright and shiny with the agony of yesterday. Yesterday, when I'd lain next to Dad's still body for close to an hour while the requisite phone calls were made, and my parents' pastor arrived to sit with us, praying and reading in his lilting Scottish accent passages from scripture meant for comfort that only made me sadder—"And God shall wipe away all tears from their eyes; and there shall be no more death, neither sorrow, nor crying, neither shall there be any more pain." Yesterday, when two mild men in dark suits came from the funeral home, and I'd let go of my beloved dad's hand for the final time. Yesterday, when I'd watched the same men wheel a stretcher that carried an emaciated form, shrouded in a black, zippered bag, out the front door of our house, load it into a hearse, and drive away.

Our little disoriented group moved through the crowded passageway and up the escalator. We went directly to a small, upscale women's boutique on the third floor where Mom had shopped a few times before. As soon as we walked in, a middle-aged saleswoman folding a stack of cashmere sweaters behind the counter smiled broadly and said, "Merry Christmas! Can I help you find anything?" There were no other shoppers in the store, so she was prepared to give us her full attention.

Michael answered for all of us, "Just browsing right now," his tone a definitive command for her to keep her distance.

She didn't take the cue. Her smile widened, and when she moved to where we were half-heartedly sifting through clothes on a nearby rack, her high heels making tiny clicks on the floor, it was clear she would not be deterred from the possibility of a sale. "I've just hung up some new arrivals over here that would be fantastic pieces for a holiday party! What are we shopping for?"

Mom gripped my hand, and the anguished, bewildered look on her face sprung me to action.

"My mom has an event this weekend," I said to the saleswoman, deciding to harness her eagerness to move what now seemed like an ill-conceived process along more quickly. "She needs something dressy, but not too flashy." I didn't tell her the whole truth, and no one else did either, so I left it at that.

"I'm sure we'll find the perfect thing," she said and turned to my mother. "Are you looking for a dress? Pants and a pretty top?"

Mom's brow creased as she tried to dissect the question, and she looked about ready to cry. She had no idea what she was looking for.

"Maybe a skirt?" I suggested and gently directed Mom to a stool that rested against the wall.

"With a nice blazer?" Ellen chimed in. Ellen had excellent fashion sense. She was one of those people who seemed always put together with style that appeared effortless. She followed the saleswoman over to another rack, her tacit mission to preview some options and limit the choices.

When Mom emerged from behind the long cloth curtain of the dressing room wearing a knee-length pencil skirt and a fitted black watch plaid jacket, she stood in front of the mirror, smoothing her hands down the front of the jacket and peered uncertainly at her image. The outfit was elegant and fit her beautifully. The saleswoman, too-cheerful still, couldn't stop gushing about how perfect the ensemble was. "And it's so wonderfully versatile," she said more than once.

Mom turned to us. "What do you think?" Beneath her hesitant words I heard the real question: *Is this the kind of a thing a widow wears?*

"Get it," we urged before she had the chance to scrutinize the tags and protest the lofty prices that surpassed what she typically spent on clothing. "Dad would love it," Mark said.

Mom's eyes filled, and she ducked back into the dressing room before the saleswoman noticed. In my mind, I saw a fleeting image of my dad, a slow smile stretching across his face, a quick nod signaling his approval. As quickly as the image came, it was gone, and I felt only the deepening void of separation that opened when the hearse disappeared over the hill at the top of my parent's street.

I couldn't stand being in this store anymore, and I escaped through the open door to wait in the hallway while my brothers helped Mom pay for her purchases. I breathed in a gulp of air and leaned against the cool metal railing, staring down at the noisy confusion that filled the two floors below me. Crowds of people bustled in and out of stores.

The ring of their laughter and boisterous prattle hurt my ears. How was it possible that none of them knew what had happened? I wanted to tell them and make them take notice. To scream: "My dad died!" into the open space in front of me for everyone to hear. It didn't make sense, all this momentum. But I felt it happening anyway—the moving forward. I felt myself unwillingly being swept up with it. Away from yesterday, away from all the days before yesterday. All the days where Dad was. I didn't want to be here where he *wasn't.* To travel ahead into all the moments where he would never be.

Mom appeared with the rest of my siblings in the boutique's doorway, a garment bag hanging over one arm, a shopping bag clutched in her other hand. She paused and blinked, adjusting her eyes from the dimness of the shop to the natural light filtering through the windows above. I reached out and took the shopping bag from her hand. Mirrored on everyone else's face was the same desperation that I felt to flee this place. We hurried back down the two flights of escalators.

As we maneuvered through the merry-making herd and neared the exit doors, I recognized a figure approaching from the opposite direction and breathed a small gasp. Pulling her heavy winter coat around her plump body was Patty, the kind and funny palliative care nurse who'd made weekly visits to the house for the last six weeks to help monitor my father's meds; who'd been with us the day before he died. She stopped, and a flicker of surprise crossed her features. Then she flashed a wry smile, and said, "Look! It's the mourners."

Mourners. The word took hold of something that was already growing inside of me, concretizing a new identity.

"We're shopping!" I blurted. I held up the bag in my hands to offer further proof.

"Yes, you are," Patty said. She didn't have to say anything more. She stepped forward to hug my mother. The rest of us squeezed in, a communal relief welling up in us, as we each reached for a slice of reassurance from the one person in the crowd who, in this interrupted moment when everything seemed wrong, saw us for who we were.

The Weasel
Friday

MY FEET ACHED. The chunky heels I was wearing were fashionable but impractical for long periods of standing. My right temple throbbed and signaled a developing migraine, not my first this week.

The steady queue of visitors coming through the white, paneled doors of Snow's Funeral Home seemed to be dwindling. I glanced at the clock on the wall. 6:45. It was almost over. The visitation that started at 4 officially ended at 7. Our original receiving line had disbanded about a half hour ago. Now, my three brothers, my two sisters-in-law, my dad's sisters, and their spouses clustered in small groups chatting with family friends in hushed voices. Since Dad was being (or had been?) cremated, there was no casket. No body to view. Instead, the displays of photos on easels positioned around the room created gathering points. I'd steered clear of them for most of the evening, but even when I was not looking, I could see Dad smiling out from the curated snapshots of vacations, holidays, graduations, weddings. My family's history. A history that had come to a sudden halt thirty-six hours earlier.

I searched the room for Mom. She was at the other end with her sisters and our pastor. Someone had made her sit. She leaned her head against the back of the upholstered chair. Her eyes were puffy and blank, her face tired. I was glad she was off her feet. She needed rest. A nonstop parade of people from all facets of our lives had filed through the room tonight to express their condolences. Lifelong friends who drove three hours to be here from Moncton, the hometown we'd left

234

ten years ago after Dad's surgery; former patients from Dad's general practice and surgical days; colleagues from the law firm that housed Dad's Canadian Medical Protective Agency office in Halifax; congregants from my parents' church; neighbors; some local friends of mine; many of David's. Younger than the rest of us by five years, he'd lived in Halifax with Mom and Dad the longest.

A few minutes ago, a tall, gray-haired gentleman I didn't recognize had walked over and shook my hand. "I own the Irving station on the Bedford Highway," he'd said, stuffing his hands back into the pockets of his ill-fitting dress pants and shifting his weight from one foot to the other. David had worked there pumping gas on weekends when he was in high school. "I was so sorry to hear what had happened. Your dad was a very kind man. He always thanked me for washing his windshield."

I wasn't used to having our family story on display, and I felt uncomfortable in my skin. I was tired. Tired of hearing people's well-intentioned words that often included, "I wish I'd known about your dad sooner." Tired of smiling in response and reassuring, "Almost no one knew." Tired of the damned heels. Chris stood beside me, chatting with my friend Yolanda. She'd been helping me remember the names of church people I should know but couldn't seem to keep straight. I was about to excuse myself to the bathroom when another man from church approached. This one I did know, though not by his real name. We called him the Weasel.

The nickname presumably came from Dad after some interaction they'd had and it stuck. The guy's slicked back hair, his tailored suits and cheap ties, and his too-good-to-be-true greased and polished finish made me recoil at his approach.

Using his role as a church elder to weasel his way into the privacy of my dad's final days, he'd called daily for status updates. "To report to the church's prayer chain," he claimed, self-righteousness oozing from his voice. "To give the prayer warriors the specifics they need." I knew better. I knew he was vying to be the first to broadcast the news of my dad's death to the rest of the congregation.

I fielded most of the calls. He was never satisfied when I told him that Dad's condition was deteriorating. "What does that mean, Melanie?" he asked. "What does that look like?" I gripped the phone receiver until my fingers hurt to keep from screaming, "It looks like he's dying, you idiot!"

The day before Dad died, the Weasel phoned and said that God had spoken to him. I was always suspicious of people who reported having a direct line.

"I feel called to come with the other church elders and anoint your dad and pray for healing. When would be a good time?"

I imagined the indignity of the Weasel and his cohorts circling my dad's bed and praying for healing while he was so obviously dying. I'd prayed for healing since I was thirteen. Please, please, please, I'd begged. Healing that wasn't coming. I didn't need to consult with the rest of the family before responding to the Weasel's request. "I'm sorry," I said, marshalling my best reverent voice. "It seems God is telling you something different than what we are hearing here. God's telling us it's time for my dad's suffering to be over. That's what we are praying for now."

I hung up the phone.

Now, as he approached me two days later, I had no escape. He leaned in to hug me. I clenched my teeth and weakly hugged him back. "Thank you for coming," I said. My standard opener for the evening.

"Your dad's story has been such an inspiration to us," he said, keeping his hand resting on my arm. My skin bristled beneath it. I struggled not to shake it off. "He was such a Godly example of Christian strength." I nodded and tried to figure out how to kick Chris to tell him I needed rescuing.

The Weasel looked into my eyes, then turned his own toward the ceiling, a sanctimonious smile curving his lips, and said, "Don't you feel the presence of the Lord right now?"

I wanted to spit in his face.

My dad was dead. Dead. I was twenty-three years old, and I was standing at my father's wake. *My father.* My favorite person. Ever. My fifty-three-year-old father was dead. Gone. Disappeared. I'd watched him disappear for ten years as the disaster of AIDS—its stigma, its cruelty—destroyed him. I was standing at my father's wake politely accepting the sympathy of people who had no clue what we'd endured. The secret. The isolation. The loneliness. The agony of the unknown. I couldn't stop seeing the black, zippered bag, slowly wheeled out of our house. And every time the kind funeral director ducked his head into this room to make sure everything was going smoothly, I wanted to beg him to tell me where Dad's body was now. Was it here? Somewhere beneath my feet? Waiting? To be burned? My mind churned with horrific images of flames and melting flesh. My dad was dead and nothing made sense.

On Wednesday night, I'd crept into David's bedroom and sat on the edge of his bed. My eighteen-year-old brother whispered into the darkness, "I'm too young not to have a dad." I was twenty-three years old, and I was too young not to have Dad.

My dad was dead.

How could God possibly be present in any of this?

I stared at the Weasel.

"Do I feel the presence of the Lord?" I stepped away from his touch, out of reach. I choked on a bitter laugh. "No," I replied, watching his pious smile falter. "I don't."

Doubts
Saturday

EVERYONE STARED FROM the pews behind me when I rose to the first chords of the hymn, "Great is Thy Faithfulness," as they echoed through the bright, open sanctuary of my parents' church. I fought the desire to look back and see who else was there. My hands smoothed my skirt, soothed by the soft velvet despite my general disdain for what I was wearing. After we'd taken Mom shopping for her outfit, she'd urged me to buy something new, saying, "Dad would have wanted it." So, I grudgingly made the trip to another boutique in downtown Halifax with my sister-in-law Yvonne. Unable to make any decisions for myself, I let a pushy saleswoman talk me into buying this getup: a long floral, velvet skirt in muted tones of burgundy, black, and gray; a fitted burgundy jacket over a crisp white blouse that buttoned to my neck. Nothing I would ever have chosen on my own. A pricey outfit I knew for certain I would never wear again. I shifted from one heeled foot to the other wishing I'd opted for something different. Something comfortable. I craved comfort.

Sunlight from the large windows on both sides of the church lit the room. Chris stood on my left, my mother to my right. Lining the remainder of the wooden pew were my three brothers, aunts, uncles, cousins. An uncommon merger of family from all sides traveling here from across Canada and the US. My cousin Stephen from Cincinnati, whom I hadn't seen for at least a decade, dashed in just as we were entering the sanctuary and joined the procession of family next to his

238

mother, my dad's oldest sister, Doreen, whose husband had taken ill and was unable to travel. Stephen managed to get a last-minute same-day flight to make it to the service. We would find out later that he kept a taxi waiting in the church parking lot with the meter running so he could go straight back to the airport.

Voices around me sang in unison: "Great is thy faithfulness, Oh God my father; / There is no shadow of turning with thee." I couldn't open my mouth. A lump had started in my throat when Chris' parents, classically trained musicians, stood and sang, "All Hail the Power of Jesus' Name." In the five years I'd known them, I'd never heard them sing together, and the powerful blend and resonance of their voices throughout the sanctuary gave me chills. The lump settled as I listened to beautiful tributes to my dad from two of his dear friends and his sister Shirley. Then, representing the rest of us, Michael spoke, bravely maintaining his composure until the very end of the eulogy we'd helped him write, when he said, "Perhaps to sum up what I'm trying inadequately to say is this: Dad was the person we most wanted to be like. Dad is still the person that we all want to be like. On Tuesday, as he was preparing to die, Mom held his hand, and through her tears she said, 'He was so good to me.'" Michael's voice caught on these words and he faltered, swallowing hard and holding tighter to the podium before finishing. "Dad was good to all of us."

Now, all I wanted to do was put my head in my hands and sob. Clamping my jaw down, I stared straight ahead and met Dad's gentle gaze from the large black and white photograph mounted on a stand at the front of the church. He was sitting on a large rock, the center of a pristine nature scene. In the background: rippling water, tall trees, a wooden rowboat. Dressed in a chambray, buttoned shirt, sleeves rolled to his elbows resting on faded blue jeans, he was smiling and relaxed—comfortable. "Sing, Mel," I heard his voice. "I love this hymn. Sing it!"

When Dad recognized that the dying part was underway, he made practical preparations. The house and cars were paid off, finances settled, my mom taken care of. He also gave a few specific requests for how he wanted to be memorialized. He asked for "Great is Thy

Faithfulness" to close the service. It was his favorite hymn. He'd played it so often on the piano over the years that I knew it by heart. The words brought him enduring comfort: "Thou changest not, thy compassions they fail not; / As thou hast been, thou forever wilt be."

They'd played this same hymn at the conclusion of my grandfather's funeral when my dad was seventeen. I imagined Dad sitting in a pew like this one in the Baptist church of his youth in Moncton, New Brunswick. The church where his father had been pastor. Dad had come home from his studies at McGill University in Montreal. The new tie he wore felt too tight at his neck. Flanked by his three older sisters and his mother, he was fighting his own battle for composure as the music began. Though the youngest in the family, he had always been their source of strength. They followed his lead. He willed his voice to work, and he harmonized the tenor notes joining the rest of the voices because he knew that was exactly what his father would want.

Now, here I was, twenty-three years old, suffering a similar scene.

"Sing, Mel," I heard again. I sucked in air, reached for my mother's trembling hand, squeezed, and lifted my voice on the final verse: "Strength for today and bright hope for tomorrow, / Blessings all mine with ten thousand beside! / Great is thy faithfulness! / Great is thy faithfulness! / Morning by morning, new mercies I see: / All I have needed, thy hand hath provided— / Great is thy faithfulness, Lord, unto me!"

I'd claimed these truths my entire life. I'd prayed. I'd lived according to Christianity's rules: I'd loved God. I'd loved my neighbor. I'd believed in the power of forgiveness—for me, for others. I'd embraced the beautiful image of heaven, a place without pain. Today, though, my dad was dead. And tomorrow, after driving the fifty miles to the country cemetery in Kennetcook, we would bury what remained.

Was God faithful? Did God care about me? Was bright hope waiting for Dad when he took that last breath?

I looked again at Dad's face smiling from the photograph. All of the certainty of faith I'd carried with me to that moment felt like it was slipping away. The only thing I knew for sure was that I sang these words because Dad asked me to.

Finale

Sunday

COLD FOUND OPENINGS in my woolen coat. At my wrists. My neck. My knees. Snuck its way in to grip my already rigid body. A thin path shoveled through deep, crusty snow led us past the white-sided country church. Past the tops of stone markers that rose from drifted mounds. Stone markers for the grave of my paternal grandfather—including the carved name of my still-living grandmother—and the graves of her parents. The sun, distant in a pale blue sky, refused us warmth. My brothers, mother, aunts, uncles, and I walked, single-file. Our faces were chafed, burned by wind. A silent line of family, we trailed behind the kind minister who carried the cherrywood box. Yesterday at Dad's service there were so many words—words to remember: Loving. Committed. Generous. Funny. Words to honor: Brilliant. Compassionate. Humble. Today, there was only the cherrywood box filled with dust. A life so large. A box so unbearably small. Our boots crunched on frozen grooves in a rhythm of resignation and did all the talking. In gloved hands, we carried long-stemmed, blush roses. Their petals rebelled against the frigid air and curled inward, dying too. We reached a shallow hole dug out from solid earth. We circled the spot. We leaned into each other and waited. The minister bent, set the box in the hole. He straightened, and with a voice unsteadied by gusty wind and emotion, said, "Peace, I leave you. My peace I give to you." I stopped listening. Tears froze on my cheeks. There was no peace as we filed past the hole. No peace as one by one, we rested our roses on the cherrywood box. No peace. Only cold, cold, cold. We did not linger. There was nothing left to do.

FAITH WOUNDS

I have come into deep waters,
where the floods overflow me.
I am weary with my crying.
My throat is dry.
My eyes fail,
looking for my God.

PSALM 69: 2-4

Turning Away
2014

THE GRAVEL PATH led me down the grass-tufted hill toward the water. The faint light of early morning made it hard to see where my sneakered feet landed. I stumbled and slowed my pace. My breath was ragged, and my heart pounded. For the past few mornings since arriving for my MFA residency—a writing program I'd started a year and a half earlier—I'd run along Main Street in Brunswick, Maine. I'd passed this park each time, but today was the first time I'd veered off the road and approached the water.

The rippling current of the Androscoggin River flowed through the tranquility of a new day with a soothing rhythm. A rocky outcropping stretched to its center. A great blue heron, a bird sometimes seen in the Christian tradition as a symbol of Christ, rested on a jagged ledge, unmoving and stately. Hints of pink and orange tinted the gray horizon heralding the sun that was still hidden behind the dark silhouettes of trees on the opposite bank. I leaned against a large rock that sat at the grass's edge above the narrow, pebbled beach. Beads of sweat dripped down my face and neck, the unseasonable humidity oppressive even at this early hour. My breathing slowed. I felt the pull to rest. To be still.

I was worn out. Not just from the four miles I'd covered on my run, but from the preceding days of workshops and seminars in which all of my focus was on my writing—writing that was taking me back to places I hadn't been for a long time, zipping me into the skin of a person I hadn't been for a long time.

The fiery ball of sun crept over the tree line and released rays of red and gold across the sky. As its warmth touched my skin, I leaned my head back, closed my eyes and let the place, the moment, swathe me in peace. *God is here.* The assertion came unbidden to my mind.

Nature had always been the place where God's presence felt most real. Standing at the summit of a mountain trail, looking across a colorful expanse of trees adorned in the brilliant colors of fall; lulled by the rhythms of the wind and churning tidal waves of the ocean; breathing in the sweet scent of spring rain as it hits the pavement; awash in the serenity of a forest blanketed in newly fallen snow; warmed by the breathtaking beauty of the sun rising over water, I could easily hang on to the belief in God at work in the symmetry and synchronicity of the natural world.

I'd been avoiding God for a long while. The process of unraveling the threads that stitched the history of Dad's illness and death had stirred up in me profoundly conflicted feelings toward God, toward the church establishment, toward so many Christians and their complicity in perpetuating the stigma of AIDS—the stigma that kept my father silent about his struggle, kept the rest of us silent. And left me so alone.

As faith abandoned me, I abandoned it.

But this morning, far away from my regular life, from the confines and people of church, I felt God. And I felt like God might be there just for me. No one else was around. No one else was experiencing this stunning sunrise. No one else was listening to this rippling water. No one else was watching this blue heron in its regal pose.

What was I supposed to do? The beauty pierced me. From a place within me, a place so dark, so bruised, so raw, a yearning to say something welled up. I felt the words burning the back of my throat. These words were ugly. Too ugly. I clamped my jaw shut, but the accusations pressed against my lips.

I thought you loved me.

I did everything you asked me to do.

How could you let this happen?

Why him?

Why me?
Where the hell were you when I needed you most?
I hate you.

These words didn't belong here. They didn't suit the splendor of this morning. The quiet of this place. How could I talk to God here when what I had to say felt so vile and contrary to what I was looking at? I bent down and picked up a handful of stones. I wanted to hurl them at the scene before me as though it was a screen that could be altered. Battered. Torn. If God could just show up a little less lovely, maybe then I wouldn't feel so out of place with the churning emotions. The doubts. Maybe then I could say some of those ugly words out loud.

I opened my palm and the stones dropped to the ground. I swallowed my words. I popped my earbuds back in and hit play on my iPod, welcoming the blaring notes of U2 and the soulful timbre of Bono's voice, singing, "But I Still Haven't Found What I'm Looking For."

How It Could Have Been Different

"YOU KNOW WHAT I keep coming back to?" Dr. B said, uncrossing his legs and repositioning himself in his chair. His forehead creased with the intensity of his thought. "I keep coming back to that pastor. The one your dad tried to talk to."

"Yeah," I said, hugging my arms close and folding a little at the waist into my protective posture. Lately, we'd been venturing into the volatile territory of faith. The most difficult territory to navigate because of my general disillusionment. But even when I determined to, I couldn't fully abandon it. Despite my dismissal, I felt a pull to try to resolve things. The figuring out part was perilous therapy ground.

Dr. B kept going. "I'd sort of like to punch that guy in the face."

He feigned shame and took an exaggerated look around the small office as though someone else might have overheard him. Talk of punching pastors was not typically understood as the "good Christian behavior" we had both been taught in our strikingly similar faith backgrounds, but he was not apologetic. His late father was a Baptist minister. He grew up in the evangelical world—a place you have to have lived to know. In our second session, when I'd recognized a familiar logo on the coffee mug he was drinking from, I'd discovered that we'd both graduated (eighteen years apart) from Gordon College, a non-denominational, Christian liberal arts school on Massachusetts' North Shore.

I also knew from small anecdotes he'd shared that faith had not been an effortless path for him either. He'd encountered his own periods of disillusionment, so an ease had emerged in our work together over the past three years that made it okay for us to say what we meant, shocking or not, appropriately "Christian" or not. And though he was using the bluntness of this statement about punching the pastor to allow space for my anger, an authentic part of him meant exactly what he said.

I smiled even though I felt like crying. Gratitude draped over me, and I loosened my arms. "I know the feeling," I said.

We'd been moving cautiously into conversations about how the Christian, particularly evangelical, response to AIDS early on—the intolerance, the bigotry, the turning of backs, the hateful messages from powerful evangelical leaders—was such a critical factor in how isolated I felt when my dad was sick. A factor that tied to my doubts about whether there was a place for God in my life now.

The story of this pastor was one I'd told Dr. B a long time ago, and I was moved, not simply because he would contemplate punching this guy on my behalf, but because he'd earmarked this event as significant enough to hold in his memory. It was a story that I only learned about long after the fact when I'd sat alone reading the manuscript of my parents' book in my basement room in Halifax. A story that I wished I had the power to rewrite because its outcome solidified a trajectory that, twenty-five years later, landed me on this couch.

Here are the facts as I know them from three stark paragraphs in The Book: On a Sunday afternoon in 1987, two years after his diagnosis, Dad was home alone and struggling with vivid thoughts of suicide. He called the pastor of the large, downtown church we attended and asked for an urgent meeting. The pastor agreed, came to our home, and my father disclosed to him the secret of his HIV infection and his anguish. The pastor offered a short prayer and then made an abrupt exit, leaving my father alone without counsel or support. The pastor later called my mother and told her that if she and my father needed his help, he would like them to come to his office so he would not have to visit them in their home.

They never heard from the man again.

Here's the scene that I can't stop imagining: My dad opens our front door. He's dressed in pleated khakis and a blue, button-down shirt. His shoulders slouch, his face is pale and drawn. With a smile that doesn't reach his pained eyes, Dad welcomes the pastor. "Thanks for coming," Dad says and clears his throat.

The pastor, popular and charismatic, dressed in jeans, sneakers, and a collared shirt, smiles broadly and claps my dad on the arm as he steps inside. "Anytime," he says. "Anytime."

Dad ushers him from the foyer to the adjacent living room and offers him a cup of coffee. The pastor accepts and sits in the armchair against the wall. Dad sinks down on the neighboring couch, looking over the pastor's shoulder at a painting of a stormy sea on the opposite wall.

"What can I do for you?" the pastor says, taking a sip of coffee from the mug Dad gives him, opening up the floor.

Folding his fingers together to steady their trembling, Dad swallows. He leans his elbows on his thighs. His heart pounds, and he feels the threat of tears pushing behind his eyes. He looks down at the tan carpet and tries to create some definable order out of the chaotic thoughts in his head. When he begins, his words are stilted and hesitant. "We are dealing with some difficult circumstances," Dad says.

At this point, I imagine the pastor leans in, his face awash with concern, his eyebrows raised.

Dad takes a breath, makes a decision, and lets the tale spill from his lips. It must take a while. There's so much to tell. As he speaks, his shoulders relax, his hands loosen. The telling itself offers him some semblance of relief.

I try to picture what the pastor is doing as Dad speaks. Does he listen closely at first? Does he look Dad in the eye? Does his demeanor change when the letters HIV/AIDS enter the room? Does the color drain from his face? Does he recoil in his chair? Does he stare for a moment at the mug in his hands before rushing to set it down on the coffee table? Does he retrace his entrance and try to remember if he shook my father's hand? I assume he does all of these things, but maybe I'm wrong.

He knows how to perform, this pastor. He's revered for his dynamic preaching from the pulpit. So maybe he manages to maintain an outward composure. Maybe he even manages to position the right look of compassion on his face when Dad reveals how despondent he feels. How he can't stop thinking that killing himself might be a better option than living with the paralyzing fear of an unclear and unlikely future with AIDS. Maybe this guy even squeezes out a tear or two of his own when Dad's flow unchecked down his cheeks.

"I don't know what to do," Dad whispers. "Where is God? Where is God in any of this?" I hear the desperation in his words. The admitted defeat.

He waits for the pastor to reach across the space between them in support. Memories of his own minister father's deep compassion and gift for spiritual counseling play in his mind. He waits for the pastor to say something. Anything.

I wonder how long it takes for Dad to realize his mistake. To feel the cold indifference filling the air. To recognize he is being rejected.

Is it when the pastor bows his head dramatically and says, "Let's pray," without expressing any feelings of his own about the tragedy he's just heard? Is it during the actual prayer, when stock phrases the pastor uses like "The mystery of your plan" and "Peace beyond all understanding" and "Thy will be done" echo through the room but do nothing to soothe Dad's wounds? Is it when the pastor says, "Amen," stands quickly, and with a series of excuses and a cursory goodbye, rushes out the door?

I picture Dad then, left alone in the living room, the shock of the pastor's sudden departure setting in. He watches through the front window as the car backs out of the driveway and disappears down the street. He stares out at the deserted street for a long time, and then drops his head into his hands.

"What a terrible missed opportunity," Dr. B said softly.

I couldn't look at him because the compassion I knew I'd see on his face might break through to the pain that lived in this story, this one and so many others like it when "God's people" couldn't have acted less godly. Pain I didn't want to face today, or any day. Instead, like I often did, I looked past his right shoulder out the window and watched the cotton-ball clouds drift lazily across the visible tract of blue sky.

"The whole story could have changed," I whispered and felt wet on my cheeks, dripping off the edge of my chin. I said the next part with certainty. "Everything would have been different."

My father was a proud man. He was used to being the guy in charge. The one always in control. Nothing would have been riskier for him than being in that position of vulnerability that day with the pastor. So exposed. When I try to imagine the courage it took for him to pick up the telephone that Sunday afternoon, I feel a clenching fist in the pit of my stomach. And when I think about that moment of rejection, picture that pastor turning away from Dad's obvious torment, a disappointment bigger than any other threatens to strangle me.

Because that was the one shot. The one shot to prove that Dad's fears of being ostracized by those around us—ostracized by those in the Christian community—were wrong. The one shot to break through the loneliness of this terrible secret and get the support that he needed. That we all needed.

"I want you to tell me the guy's name," Dr. B said, uncharacteristic anger sharpening his words as he spun his platinum wedding band around and around the knuckle of his ring finger. He then reconsidered. "But don't tell me his name because, like I said, I could punch him."

I brushed back my hair as I pressed my palm against the throbbing in my forehead and straightened. "Oh, I can tell you his name," I spat out, surprising myself with this burst of venom, "and I can tell you exactly where he is. He's been the senior pastor of one of New York City's biggest churches for the last seventeen years. I could contact him in a heartbeat."

"What would you say?"

I hesitated, a cyclone of thoughts and emotions roaring through my head. I pulled a random one from the chaos.

"Did I tell you I used to babysit his kids?" I twisted the tissue I held into a tight ball. "His three kids. I babysat for them occasionally, even after this happened with my dad." For the first time, I tried to wrap my understanding around this incomprehensible fact. My parents left the church because they couldn't reconcile this man's words from the pulpit with his behavior toward them, a hypocrisy that felt intolerable to them. They started attending a church closer to our home. But because they never explained their reasoning to me, I stayed. I kept going to youth group and worship services on Sunday night. Throughout my high school years, that downtown church was my social hub. Unaware of the pain he'd inflicted on my parents, I trusted this man's leadership and embraced his ideals, despite the nagging questions that his message couldn't answer. I went to his home. I took care of his kids. And this pastor, *my* pastor, never said anything to me. Not one thing. "What kind of person says nothing to a teenage girl who is dealing with such a devastating situation?" I asked Dr. B.

"Maybe an asshole?" Dr. B said, giving me the same sheepish look from earlier. I smiled again. I liked these rare moments when he swore. They were oddly reassuring.

The good-girl me wanted to give the pastor the benefit of the doubt. To extend him some grace. Was it unfair for me to stack the outcome of our story squarely on one man's shoulders? 1987 was a scary time when it came to AIDS. I'd lived the history. No one seemed to know the right way to respond. There was so much ignorance. So much mystery connected to this illness that took the lives of so many. Maybe I could forgive him. I had been scared then too.

A few years earlier, after recounting this story for the first time to Dr. B, I'd gone home, sat down at my laptop, and typed the man's name into the Google search bar. His bio on the New York City church's website was the first thing to pop up. When I clicked on the link, his face appeared at the top of my screen. It took me a moment to recognize him: he was bald and sported a trendy goatee and dark rimmed glasses. But I knew his face and my stomach seized. I scrolled through the site and read about his work and the impact he'd had on his congregation.

I read about his family. Those kids I used to babysit were married now with children of their own. He was somebody's grandfather.

So, I wanted to excuse him. I wanted to believe that he simply hadn't been equipped with the proper tools for the unique nature of my dad's situation. I wanted to chalk it up as one bad blip on the broader screen of his successful ministry. He was the good guy in so many other people's stories. I wanted to stop thinking that everything he'd done since 1987 was negated because of one mishandled incident.

But I couldn't.

I couldn't because in the thirty years since he'd turned his back on my dad, on my whole family, he'd never looked back. Never apologized. Never questioned his behavior enough to clarify or remedy it. Dad died, but the rest of us didn't. We were there the whole time, coping with the grief, railing against the loss. And some of us still felt the pain and confusion and loneliness of that experience as deeply as we did then. Maybe more so.

Because of this pastor and others like him, some of us struggled so hard to trust in the possibility that there were good, Christian people with good intentions, that even when they sat right in front of us, even when they set their unwavering gaze on the messiness of our doubts and questions and anger and doubted and questioned and got angry with us, even when they expressed an inclination to punch the same people we wanted to so we wouldn't feel quite so alone, we kept expecting them to turn away.

"That's what I'd say to him." I looked Dr. B in the eye. My tone was definitive even though my voice was trembling. "I'd say he's an asshole."

Grateful? It Wasn't a Gift.
1992

I WAS LATE. Arts in Concert, the first-year core fine arts class in which I was a teaching assistant, included a slide show depicting famous paintings. Packing up the projector and returning the slide carousel to the art department across campus took longer than I'd planned for. The gym was crowded and noisy when I entered, and I was out of breath. Chitchat and laughter bounced off the walls and parquet floor and reverberated through the open room. I ran my student ID through the card scanner a minute shy of being counted as tardy. Weekly attendance to Friday convocation at Gordon was mandatory, and we were granted only a few skips a semester. I'd maxed mine out.

I scanned the sea of folding chairs and looked for my roommate. I was hoping her class had dismissed early and she was saving me a seat. Sherri waved from a row near the front. I hurried down the aisle and slipped in beside her with an appreciative smile just as the college president stepped to the microphone of the wooden podium centered on the portable stage at the front of the gymnasium. He began with a few cursory announcements and then introduced the woman who would deliver the keynote convocation address of the day. Still trying to gather my thoughts after the rush to get here on time, I was only half-listening when the words "contracted HIV from a dirty needle in 1987" made me sit straighter in my chair and give him my full attention.

I stared at the small woman standing beside the president. She was maybe thirty, but her hardened features and the worn look in her eyes

254

made it difficult to tell for sure. She was dressed in a simple, knee-length skirt and white, short-sleeved top. Her thin arms, inked with tattoos, hung at her sides as she waited for her turn to speak. She curled her hands into fists and then released them in a repetitive pattern.

The walls of the gym felt like they were closing in. The anticipation of what might come in this woman's address filled me with dread. Only a handful of trusted friends here at school knew of my dad's illness. I squeezed my hands together to stop their shaking as she began to talk. I focused my eyes on the retracted basketball hoop over her head.

Her voice was husky, clearly a smoker's. "I had a tough childhood," she said. She proceeded to deliver a testimony: a narrative journey of a life that began in an abusive home, spiraled into drug use in her teens, and eventually left her homeless on the streets of Boston in her twenties. "One night, when I was at my lowest, I met this wonderful woman at a soup kitchen, and she invited me to church. I found God. For the first time in my life, things began to make sense." She talked about the rehab program that helped her get sober and start making positive changes in her life.

"And then I discovered I was HIV positive," she said, a quiver stuttering her words. "When I lived on the streets, I was desperate for drugs, and I got them however I could. We didn't really know about AIDS then, and sharing needles was the norm."

I winced, thinking of the others who might still be wandering those streets, unaware of the death sentence circulating through their bodies. Sherri rested a hand on my arm. She knew about Dad. I couldn't look at her.

I looked instead at the rapt faces of the other students around me. They hung on the woman's words and some nodded in appreciation. I could read their minds. They were waiting for the inevitable upswing to the testimony. The traditional climax in the narrative arc of the Christian conversion story. The inspirational part that provided the "and now it's okay because of God" message that made the prodigal parts of these stories palatable to them and their sheltered upbringings. As the speaker talked, I sensed she was headed that way. I squeezed my hands tighter and my fingernails dug into my skin. The muscles in my arms started to burn.

"Of course I was devastated at first. But you know what?" She paused, her eyes scanning the crowd, and I wondered how often she'd delivered this testimony. "Finding out I have AIDS has given my life purpose," she declared. A few soft "Amens" rippled through the audience. "I can protect other people from my fate. I can stand before you today and tell you to make better choices."

And then the triumphant clincher: "I thank God for giving me AIDS."

The audience erupted in applause. The sound vibrated through me, a sour taste filled my mouth. I was going to throw up. "I've got to go," I said to Sherri and shoved my way past the knees that blocked the row. I raced up the aisle toward the back exit of the gym.

I crashed through the door and stepped out into the blinding midday sun. I let the door slam behind me and walked rapidly down the path toward the parking lot. I pulled in deep, ragged breaths of the crisp air, trying to settle my heaving stomach. I wanted to storm back into the gym. I wanted to scream at the woman: "God didn't give you AIDS! God doesn't hand out deadly diseases like gifts!" I needed my words to be true instead of hers. If they weren't, and God gave Dad AIDS, then God was nobody I wanted to know.

Unsettled
2013

THE SUN RADIATED across the stretch of sand in front of me. Diamond sparks glistened on the wet pools remaining from the tide's receding wake. The air was cool but held promise of warming. The water was uncharacteristically calm, stretching to a point where sea and sky met and melted together in a line of bluish gray. Will and Lily ran ahead with the dog and urged him to venture into the waves. "Come on, Wally!" "Get the shell!" He nosed the rolling waves that lapped the beach's edge in their steady rhythm, crests breaking, foamy and white. He was tentative at first, but then his retriever instincts kicked in, and he jumped into the surf after the large clamshell Will tossed. Wally splashed through the salty spray and ducked his head below the surface, coming up with the shell in his mouth. He rushed back to the sand and shook his fur, showering the kids with water, wagging his tail in triumph. They darted in and out of the breakers, chasing and splashing. Their laughter carried through salty air. Chris and I walked hand-in-hand, following their footsteps. I breathed it in, and my body tried to relax into the soothing rhythm of the day.

It was Easter Sunday, a few months after I'd started my MFA program. While most Christians we knew crowded onto the wooden pews of their respective churches to celebrate the resurrection of Christ that morning, we were spending this sacred holiday an hour from home in Ogunquit, Maine, walking one of our favorite beaches. There was no new Easter dress for Lily, and Will had not been forced to don a shirt with a collar. There were no formal prayers or rituals. No sermons on the promises of redemption and eternal life. No resurrection hymns. There was only open air and an endless expanse of ocean.

A skulking guilt hampered my ability to fully appreciate the scene. My programming of how Easter was *supposed* to be observed had never included a day at the beach. Yet here we were for the second year in a row, distancing ourselves from the religious expectations we'd lived with for most of our lives.

A year and a half earlier, we'd walked away from church. Until then, we'd been entrenched in the evangelical Presbyterian congregation we'd attended for close to ten years. Chris served as a deacon, providing care and support to church members, and I was a ruling elder appointed by the congregation and publicly commissioned to serve as a leader on the church's governing board. I chaired the Missions' Committee and directed the Vacation Bible School Program. I sang in the choir, and both Chris and I volunteered regularly to help lead the weekly worship services. Will and Lily attended Sunday school and participated in youth socials and game nights. Then one day, Chris and I sent separate emails to the head of the church board, resigned from everything, and left. Not just that particular church, but church altogether. On the surface, our decision seemed as sudden as ripping off a Band-Aid in one clean swipe, and it's understandable that those who'd remained and had depended on our leadership felt betrayed. In truth, we'd finally reckoned with a question we'd been asking for too long: what are we doing here? The factors that led to our exodus had been brewing for years, lifting the Band-Aid slowly, bit by bit, tugging at one painful hair after another.

2007

"As for me and my house, *we* will serve the Lord," the middle-aged woman I knew by sight, but not name, declared in a defiant voice, wielding like a weapon the familiar passage of scripture—one Chris and I had printed on the back of our wedding program thirteen years earlier. She clutched the microphone stand and glared at the people packing the pews in front of her. I shifted on the hard wood of my seat and felt wash over me the judgment contaminating her words. As murmurs of agreement met her statement, I tasted something bitter. I glanced at Chris and knew by the furrow of his brow and the set of his jaw that he was struggling to control his emotions.

"Let's try to remain open-minded," pleaded the denominational representative, a stocky, fifty-something-year-old man who'd been tasked to mediate this meeting that would determine whether our conservative-leaning congregation would disaffiliate with the Presbyterian Church (USA). "There's room for disagreement, but the dialogue should continue." It was clear to me that the possibility for further dialogue that might offer other perspectives on the recent progressive amendments made by the denomination to its stances on a woman's right to choose and the ordination of LGBTQ+ ministers had disappeared when the woman at the mic drew the line that separated the "*real* Christians" from any of us who questioned the rigid thinking of the greater evangelical community and sought broader inclusion.

Earlier that evening, I'd entered our church's historic sanctuary feeling hopeful. I knew many of the people who filled the pews and believed they knew me. We worshipped together on Sundays. Shared meals. Got together for play dates with our kids. We met in small group settings and endeavored to study the Bible, discussing how to apply the Christian standards found in passages of scripture to our modern lives, challenging each other to keep conversations open to a variety of interpretations. We revealed painful parts of our life journeys, asking difficult questions about how God fit into the suffering and grief we encountered along the way. Four years earlier, Chris and I stood at the front of that sanctuary while the minister baptized our children—Will, two, and Lily a baby—and we made a commitment, echoed by the congregation, to faithfully guide them in their Christian formation. And we believed that this was the place to do it. As with other churches we'd attended in our life together, Chris and I bumped up against conflicting views to ours on some of the more hot-button social, and often political, issues—abortion, gay marriage, even gun control—but we believed there was room for differing opinions. We held out that the community was stronger than any of the cracks at its foundation. Because we'd both grown up in the church, had experienced it and our Christian faiths as central values in our families, it felt important for us, and our children, to be part of such a community. Though there had been rumblings of discord from some prominent church members about denominational decisions over the past few months, I'd trusted that values of compassion, mercy, tolerance, and justice were rooted in most of the congregants I knew.

But as the evening progressed, and I listened to many of these congregants espouse dogmatic stands against the direction the denomination was headed—a "holier-than-thou" posturing that quoted Biblical passages about "following in the ways of the wicked" and cited the need to uphold "traditional family values," culminating in As For Me Lady's final declaration—that trust evaporated. Conspicuously absent in any of their words was Christ's call to "love one another, as I have loved you."

I scanned the faces around me and met the eyes of a few close friends who appeared as staggered by this display as I was. Their expressions reflected the disappointment that gripped my chest, but I experienced something deeper. In that moment—even before the votes for disaffiliation were cast that would, in the following months, result in a bitter congregational split—an old wound reopened, first cut years ago when unbending stances, reminiscent of these ones, stigmatized HIV/AIDS and made it impossible for my family to seek support from those closest to us.

2009

Pleasant conversation filled the lobby and greeted Chris, Will, Lily, and me as we filed out the wooden doors at the back of the church sanctuary. The organ postlude that echoed the themes of the morning's final congregational hymn, "Guide Me, O Thou Great Jehovah," accompanied our exit. Chris and I paused to chat with a few friends while the kids went to inspect the requisite post-service snacks that garnished a table against the far wall. I felt the touch of a soft hand on my elbow and turned to see Peg, a stout woman in her seventies, standing at my side.

"I just finished your parents' book," she said, her hand still on my elbow, guiding me away from the clusters of people to a quieter spot at the base of the staircase leading to the church's second floor. "I took it out of the church library after your talk."

Six weeks earlier, on the Sunday before World AIDS Day, I'd stood trembling next to our senior pastor at the pulpit and spoken for the first time publicly about my family's experience with HIV/AIDS. In the two years since the denominational split, Chris and I had been heartened by what seemed to be a more forward-thinking and inclusive vision for this emerging church spearheaded by a new pastor and the small minority of members who'd remained part of the Presbyterian Church (USA). We'd chosen to stay with them, stepping into positions of leadership, committed to helping move that vision forward. As the newly appointed chair of the Missions' Committee, I offered to share some pieces of my family's story in the hope of broadening our congregation's awareness of the national and global impact of the AIDS pandemic and to begin a conversation about tangible ways our church might respond. "If AIDS does not have a face for you, make it mine," I said at the close of my talk. "I am someone you know whose life is forever changed by this devastating disease." A number of church members reached out to me in the weeks that followed, expressing their desire to learn more about my, and the larger, AIDS story, and I was encouraged by the positive reactions. I donated a couple of copies of The Book to the church's collection.

Now, though, faced with Peg's stony, impossible-to-read demeanor, I felt a flutter of anxiety in my stomach. She was the matriarch of the church's "first family"—members of this New England congregation for decades. Her long-term involvement in the evolution of this church over the years gave her an impression of ownership, and she was not one to hold or temper her opinions for the sake of camaraderie. Chris and I had been stunned that her family had stayed on this side of the line after the church split because most of our interactions revealed them to be quite legalistic in their theology.

"Your father was a very Godly man, a Godly man," she repeated, the hard lines of her face beginning to soften. "He was so young. Such a terrible tragedy." I nodded, unsure how to respond. She suddenly leaned in, and I saw tears behind her round, plastic-rimmed glasses. "My son died of AIDS too," she spoke in an urgent, confessional whisper. "Nobody knows."

Surprise followed by deep empathy swept through me. I reached for her hand, feeling the roughness of her skin against mine. "Oh, Peg! I'm so sorry to hear that," I said. I didn't know she'd had another child. The child I did know also went to this church and served with me on various church committees, and, like Peg, was not shy about expressing views—particularly, it seemed, when they conflicted with mine. I was not a fan. But now there was this: an intimate window into this family's history that might account for their rigid exteriors, and I felt my perspective begin to revise.

"You're fortunate you can talk about your father," Peg said, letting go of my hand, her tone recalibrating, hardening once more. "At least he can't be blamed for what happened to him. There's nothing you have to be ashamed about."

The implication of her words hit with such force that I took an involuntary step backwards. Emotion charged my body as I thought about this prodigal son who hadn't turned out the way his family wanted, his life and death unspeakable because—what? He'd had unprotected sex? He was gay? An addict?

The reality of this stigma was nothing new, especially in churches, but I'd believed that change was possible here, that minds were open to more accepting ways of thinking. And maybe they were. I searched the group of congregants milling in the lobby, the goodwill and warmth of their conversations reaching me. If my family's story were different, if I'd stood at that pulpit and talked about my father contracting AIDS by another means instead of through a blood transfusion, would that goodwill still have been extended to me?

Confronted by Peg's pained and expectant gaze, waiting for some sort of avowal of her choices, I wanted to hold compassion for the narrow borders of her ability to love her own child and acknowledge the complexities of her circumstances. But all I could register was the hierarchy she was presenting—particularly with her emphasis on my father's "Godliness"—of who deserves Jesus's love and acceptance and who doesn't. A hierarchy that continued to permeate this evangelical culture, no matter how progressive it appeared. Was change actually possible? The misgivings of the past layered beneath the misgivings of this moment, and I felt beaten.

I summoned enough energy to remain civil as I spoke the truth I felt. "I'm sorry about what happened to your son."

2010

My hand trembled as I read the contents of the letter. Sentence fragments leaped out from the page: "*a Godly perspective on missions*" "*the long-standing tradition of this church*" "*support only those organizations with a deep evangelical focus.*" My fingers clenched the edges, creasing the page. I wanted to tear it to shreds, but I couldn't because I was sitting in a pew smack in the middle of the sanctuary surrounded by my fellow Sunday morning parishioners, and the service was about to start. I was today's liturgist. These people expected poise and dignity from me. Exposing the anger boiling my blood at that moment was out of the question. I stuffed the letter into my bag along with my anger.

The organist played the final notes of the prelude, and I slid past Chris, stepped up to the pulpit, gripped its wooden sides and took a deep, calming breath before pasting on a bright smile. I looked out at the expectant faces of the congregation and declared: "This is the day that the Lord has made. Let us rejoice and be glad in it! It is my pleasure to welcome you to our church on this Sunday morning. May the fellowship of this day and the words of this service fill you with the peace and joy of our Lord Jesus Christ. Please stand and join in the songs of worship printed in your bulletin." The musicians began, and I walked back to my seat. I met the eyes of the letter's author. I set my jaw and did not look away.

His letter was a warning.

Minutes before the service, this long-time member of the congregation, a white-haired man nearing eighty, had approached me in the church lobby as I made my way toward the sanctuary entrance. He handed me a plain white envelope with the words *Just an FYI* penned in scrawling script on the front. He smiled pleasantly and said, "I thought this would help you in your role." I had no delusions. Though he was well-respected for his service to this community, his arrogant touting of his desire to hold tight to tradition in the face of change made him hard for me to like. I also sensed his disdain for women in positions of leadership. The role he alluded to when he handed me the letter was my position as chair of the church's Missions' Committee—a title he once held.

The Sunday before, feeling helpless in the wake of the catastrophic magnitude 7.1 earthquake that decimated the Caribbean nation of Haiti, I also felt compelled to provide members of our church with some resources for offering support. I included an insert in the church bulletin listing specific organizations raising funds for the relief effort. My brother Michael was the Canadian executive vice president for World Vision, one of the largest Christian international development and relief organizations, and I'd asked for his advice. "The best place to start," he told me over the phone, "is with the organizations that already have a presence in Haiti. They can provide the most effective and immediate relief." The Red Cross and World Vision were his top two picks. I'd added the Salvation Army and also the Presbyterian Disaster Relief Fund to incorporate a link to our denomination's efforts.

Only after the fact did secondhand murmurings reach me that my inclusion among the listed websites of the Red Cross, an organization without a specific Christian affiliation, had ruffled some feathers among the church's old guard—particularly this man's. His letter was a direct response. He presented a detailed account of our congregation's past missions' activities and his own dictate of where our future mission focus should be. The subtext was clear: Our primary goal should be to reach all the "lost souls" around the globe and share the "good news" of Jesus. I'd grown up with this mindset in my Baptist tradition—the "get 'em out and get 'em saved" mantra, my dad used to call it, revealing his own skepticism about the church's emphasis on converting as many people as possible at the cost of building real, authentic relationships. This was the first time I was explicitly encountering the directive in this church setting, however, and I felt immediate pushback.

I pictured the haunted face of a little girl who'd appeared in one of CNN's ongoing reports from Haiti the night before. She wasn't more than four or five. She sat in the dusty rubble outside one of the many destroyed buildings in Port-au-Prince. Her clothes were torn, her hair matted, her face dirty. My heart pitched as I'd watched her huddle beneath a filthy sheet while the rain created muddy pools around her. Her sunken, empty eyes stared straight into the camera. Her suffering was palpable.

The mandate to attach "religious strings" to aid and compassion made me feel sick. The "good news" was not what that little girl needed at this moment. She needed shelter. Food. Water. She needed a mother and a father. Weren't we called to "do justly" and "love kindness" in whatever forms they took? There was something insidious about a mindset that ordered us to approve only certain organizations, whether they were the most effective ones or not, to give those things to her. I didn't care. I only cared that she got them.

2011

My passion and vision for this church are clouded, and with that knowledge, I realize that my time of service on this board has run its course.

The final words of the letter, my resignation from the church governing board on which I'd served for a year and a half, scrolled across my laptop's screen. I read them one more time, took a shaky breath, and clicked send. As the swooshing sound signaled the departure of the outgoing message, I sat back in my rolling chair, staring at the bare, November branches of the trees out the window behind my desk. A muddled concoction of profound relief and intense grief inundated my body.

After months of indecision, I'd let go of the hope that the direction our church was headed might somehow be different than the one I'd already traveled in my life. When I accepted the invitation to become an elder, I had little idea of the existing turmoil behind the scenes involving the church leadership and staff. The backstage pass I was handed exposed a grim reality I didn't want to see: the Christian leaders we followed and entrusted with carrying out the church's vision were as flawed as anyone else.

In only my second meeting of the board, I sat stunned, clenching my seat until my knuckles hurt, as a senior staff member unraveled. A seething rage filling the person's words, etching their face as they refused to answer accusations from other staff members of dishonesty and possible abuses of power. This was someone I thought I knew, but in that moment, they were unrecognizable. I felt my foundation of security shift. Doubt seeped through the growing fissures. *It's time to get out,* a voice inside my head warned. *This is not where you want to be.* Chris was ready to walk away then, but I pushed for us to stay a while longer, clinging to the hope that I still had something to offer, a pathological need to do what was expected of me drowning out that warning voice.

Where else could we go? And what about our kids? Hadn't we promised to give them a spiritual home? I felt like I was on a cliff's edge, staring into the unknown, too afraid to trust my instincts and take flight. For my entire life, faith had been a collective act, and belonging to a church community was pivotal to my overall understanding and faith practice. As disenchantment unsteadied my security in that community, it snarled with thorny feelings toward God that I'd internalized long ago.

From the moment the catastrophe of Dad's illness struck our family, I lost my certainty in God's goodness. My Christian faith told me that God was active in my life. That God loved me. That God wanted the very best for me. Then Dad got sick and Dad died. Senselessly. Needlessly. I'd tried so hard to believe that God had been there. But looking back, I was having a hard time finding God in any of it. Searching through the ruined rooms that had housed my faith, I was having an even harder time trying to find God now.

What was left? I wondered, still staring out the window, my thoughts as murky as the overcast sky.

—

Ahead of us on the sandy beach, Will and Lily were getting bolder. They rolled their pant legs up above their knees and ventured farther into the water, jumping the cresting waves that curled into white froth. Wally scampered around them, fueled by their excitement. The water was icy. Too icy for me. I was content to walk beside Chris on sun-warmed sand. It squished beneath my toes. A sandpiper flitted in and out of the tide, its tiny feet moving at lightning speed. I wondered where it was going.

Chris spread his arms wide toward the breathtaking expanse stretching in front of us. "I can't think of a better way to spend this morning than enjoying all of this. Where else is God, if not here?"

"Don't you feel guilty that we're not in church?" I asked. I kept looking for him to mirror my conflicted feelings about our decision to step away. On purpose, I thought about it as "stepping away" instead of "leaving" because it felt less definitive, and it felt important that the action not have clear definition. Lack of definition allowed for the possibility of shifts in thinking, for the foundational elements of the Christian faith, intertwined with my family heritage, with my memories of my father, to find some meaningful space in my life.

"I don't feel guilty at all," Chris said. He didn't share my tension about our church departure. For him, it wasn't a crisis of faith. It was a faith reckoning. Unburdening himself of the expectations that no longer felt like his to meet. Recognizing that living out his faith and sharing it with our children was not contingent on sitting in a pew every Sunday morning. He was comfortable letting things be what they were in the moment. Unlike me, he did not need a definitive plan to keep moving forward. He was willing to wait and see what came next and trusted that we'd figure it out together. I trusted him, so for now, that's what I held on to.

"I just don't know how we got here." I sighed, my eyes glued to the receding water. The rhythm of the waves—rolling close, then rolling away, but always turning back again—soothed me. He put his arm around my shoulders and guided me toward the ocean's edge where the kids were splashing with Wally. "Yes," he said, "you do."

LETTING GO,
AND HOLDING ON

For whatsoever from one place doth fall,
Is with the tyde unto another brought:
For there is nothing lost, that may be found, if sought.

EDMUND SPENSER,
The Faerie Queene

Loosened Grip
2014

"You are not broken, you know."

Dr. B's statement dropped into the quiet that had been parked between us for the past few minutes. I was working on recomposing myself after dissolving into a particularly messy puddle of emotion. My face buried in my hands, my instinctual effort to hide. When Will and Lily were little, they'd cover their eyes and think that since they couldn't see us, we couldn't see them. I was hoping the trick was working on Dr. B. Even after all this time and all our work, I hated this raw exposure.

His declaration compelled me to look up, though. Despite the rush of tears flooding my cheeks, I gave a weak smile. "I'm not exactly sure what to do with that," I said.

Dr. B leaned back in his chair and smiled too, recognizing that this simple statement in the context of the intense discussion we'd been having about my family dynamics before my breakdown might seem a bit anti-climactic on the scale of grand revelations. "There it is," he chuckled. "You can thank me now, pay up, and go forth. Our work here is done."

The press of anguish I'd felt moments earlier lifted, and I managed to straighten my caved-in posture. I let my arms loosen from their grip at my waist and grabbed a tissue from the box next to me, sweeping it across my wet face.

Dr. B let the joke trail off, and his voice shifted to a more reflective tenor. "It just struck me in a way I've never thought about or verbalized before," he said, "that you don't simply think the grief you still carry is unwarranted. You truly believe it means there's something fundamentally wrong with you."

"But isn't there?" I asked. For me, it was the most obvious of answers. I'd sat on this couch nearly every week for three years manifesting some version of this same messy emotional puddle. In my conversations with Dr. B, I circled back again and again to many of the same, unresolved themes and questions that echoed in the memories of my experiences. Unable to put them down or let them go. We'd peeled back a lot of painful layers since I first walked through his door, but I didn't see my need for those conversations ending anytime soon. "Going forth" without his support was something I couldn't yet imagine. But I worried that, in spite of his kindness and ongoing reassurance, I was wearing down his patience. I worried that my endless rehashing of the same topics must be tedious for him. His inbox contained more than one of my emails saying as much. Though I might have changed "tedious" to "torture." He claimed it wasn't. I tried to believe him, but it was hard not to think that it was only a matter of time before he threw up his hands and told me there was nothing more he could do for me. I gestured to him, to the open space of his office, to my own shaky demeanor. "Isn't all of this a pretty good indicator that something's not right with me?"

Dr. B sat up straighter and brushed his hand over his balding head, then raked his fingers through the still thick hair on the side. "Did something tragic happen to you and your family? Yes. Are you traumatized? Yes. Are you struggling with the ongoing effects of that trauma? Yes. Have those struggles been more difficult for you to work through than they have been for your brothers? Possibly. But does that mean you are broken? No, it doesn't." He was thoughtful again. "Maybe that's the thing you need to start letting go of."

He'd tracked back to the place this conversation began before things got messy. I'd expressed, yet again, my wish that I could talk to my brothers—to my mother—about the things I talked to him about. "You'd think they'd be the ones who would understand it the most.

Understand *me* the most," I'd said. "But honestly? I think they'd find it all ridiculous and exhausting. Totally self-indulgent. And definitely something that needs to be fixed so I can get back to being *normal.*" I'd paused, an uncomfortable sensation of disloyalty mounting my spine. I qualified. "They wouldn't tell *me* that. They're not mean or unfeeling. They'd listen and try to understand. But I can imagine the 'concern' about my general stability that they'd be expressing to each other behind my back. And *you,*" I'd looked at Dr. B pointedly, planting a wry smile on my face. "I can hear them asking, 'What kind of quack therapist takes three years to help someone work through her grief?'"

He'd smiled, too, but then he said the thing that triggered the puddle. "You spent—what?—almost thirty years *not* working through your grief. Keeping it bottled up so deep that even you couldn't access it. When I think about that," he said softly, the compassion in his eyes so genuine it hurt, "three years of working on it doesn't seem like very long at all."

Now, as I considered his declaring me unbroken, I recognized the challenge it posed to my habitual way of thinking about myself—a way of thinking long-defined by how I positioned myself in relationship to my three brothers. Michael and Mark, older and wiser, led the way. Destined by birth order and gender, I'd followed. I tried to keep up, tried to do what they did, like what they liked, and always, always fell just a bit short. Five years after me, David arrived, gifted with a precociousness that, despite his starting position, propelled him forward in the ranks, allowed him to match, and even surpass, what the rest of us had done. No matter what I'd accomplished academically or musically—the two main bars for success in my family—the reality was that one of the boys had done it first and a little better. My successes didn't feel exceptional ("Even though they are," Dr. B. liked to remind me before reciting a litany of grade point averages, earned degrees, career successes and recognitions); they just felt expected. And when it took me longer to puzzle out the same math problems and science equations and musical notes that they'd solved with such ease, I'd repeated the same question over and over again: what's wrong with me?

I'd repeated variations of the same question here, to Dr. B, more times than I could count. Why did I hold this grief so close? Why did my wounds refuse to heal? Why did I carry this trauma everywhere when my brothers seemed to have left it somewhere behind them? Why was I so bent on remembering and documenting what everyone else seemed content to forget? Why couldn't I stop telling this story? Why couldn't I land in a resolved place with my faith—decide if God mattered to me or not and move on? Why couldn't I drop the notion that I needed to figure that answer out right now? Why was I still here in this cramped office, sitting on the same center cushion of this worn-out leather couch, desperate for this kind-eyed man in the wingback chair to tell me it was okay? What the hell was wrong with me?

In this moment, with his intent gaze meeting mine, Dr. B offered me a concrete answer: "Nothing. There's nothing wrong with you."

I looked down at my hands, suddenly self-conscious. I smoothed one thumbnail over the other in a repetitive motion. I'd done the tears for today; I didn't want to start crying again this close to the end of our appointment.

"You are different from your brothers, Melanie," Dr. B said. "You have lived this family story in a different way than they have." He pulled at the cuff of his dress shirt and straightened his jacket sleeve. "Different doesn't mean worse or better. Different doesn't mean wrong or right. Different doesn't mean bad or good. And different definitely doesn't mean broken." He gave an exaggerated shrug to his shoulders before he stood up. "Different just means different."

When I got to my car in the parking lot, I didn't immediately turn the key in the ignition. I sat for a few minutes, resting my head against the seatback, and closed my eyes. The sun that streamed through the windshield was welcome after the air-conditioned chill of the office. My mind sifted through the contents of the day's session and bounced around Dr. B's newly verbalized suggestion. What if he was right? The question thrummed against my temples, and with it, the slightest trace of something else—a rare sensation of confidence. I opened my eyes and reached for my purse on the seat beside me. I dug into its pocket and pulled out a pen and the compact, leather-bound notebook that I carried, just in case I wanted to remember something. I opened to a clean page. I scrawled *2014* in the corner, and then in large, capital letters across the center of the page, I wrote: YOU ARE NOT BROKEN. I traced the outline of each letter, bolding their edges, adding decorative swirls, making them something I wanted to look at. I pushed the pen against the paper as hard as I could without ripping it and underlined the word NOT.

Twice.

Steps Ahead

I DROPPED MY keys and purse onto the wood-topped kitchen island, adding to the clutter of mail, school papers, and dirty dishes that were already there. A loud sigh whooshed past my lips. After a hectic day of catching up on work, running errands, and taxiing the kids to school and sports, and only an hour before leaving again to pick up Lily from gymnastics, I couldn't quite face the clean-up. I turned away from the mess and kicked off my ballet flats. One slid under a stool and the other settled upside down next to the refrigerator.

Wally followed at my bare heels, his tail wagging a vigorous greeting while I padded across the hardwood floors through the kitchen and family room to the living room and pulled the window shades to insulate our world from the gathering darkness outside. It had been under an hour since I left to drop Lily off, but he welcomed me back like I'd just returned from a long trip. I didn't mind his enthusiasm.

"Who's a good dog?" I asked, my voice rising to that singsong pitch we reserved for babies and animals. Wally pushed against my calf, and I scratched behind his ears. At the front door, I flicked the switch to turn on the outside lights for Chris. He was teaching in Boston and wouldn't be home until after nine. I stopped at the base of the stairs and rested my hand on the banister.

"How's it going?" I called up to Will. I'd left him with strict instructions not to turn on the Red Sox game until he finished all his schoolwork. Wally sat at my feet. He was afraid of these stairs, and though we'd used every possible coaxing tactic to try to get him to climb up, he refused to leave the main floor.

When Will didn't answer right away, I repeated the question. "Homework done?"

"No."

It was one word, but there was a catch in his voice when he said it, and I sensed a problem.

"What's going on?" I asked, mounting the steps two at a time, hastening to where Will's open bedroom door leaked light into the dark hallway.

I was not expecting the scene that met me when I stepped into his room: My fourteen-year-old son sat cross-legged on the oatmeal-colored carpet, his back against his closet door, his new fishing rod balanced on his lap. His blond head was bent over the reel while his frenzied fingers worked at the tangled loops of clear line knotted around the mechanism. His shoulders shook and ragged sobs escaped his mouth. He lifted his blotchy face to look at me; a mess of tears and snot streaked his cheeks. His thick-lashed blue eyes were puffy and panicked.

"I think I broke it," he moaned when I dropped down to my knees beside him. His fingers didn't pause in their frantic efforts to fix the snagged reel.

"Oh, buddy," I said, his overt distress drawing tears to my eyes and making my chest cave a little. I wrapped one arm around his heaving shoulders and placed my other hand over his hand to stop its movement. Our hands were the same size. His fingers shook under my grip. "Let me take a look."

Fishing was trending among the adolescent boys in our neighborhood. With a certain Huck Finn-esque quality, Will and his friends rode their bikes to a nearby pond, fishing poles protruding from their backpacks, and spent free afternoon hours casting lines for largemouth bass and pickerel.

Delighted to see Will's growing love for one of my dad's favorite pastimes, my mother jumped at the idea of buying him a rod for his birthday. Until then, he'd been borrowing an old one from his friend Jack. Will had devoted the last two days since his birthday to organizing and reorganizing for his next expedition, the clear, slotted tackle box we'd given him that contained various lures and baits, hooks, floats, small pliers and scissors.

Will was not a kid who asked for a lot, but he developed a lasting affection for the things he had. Besides the expected team trophies from soccer and baseball that adorned the rooms of most boys his age, his shelves held other little treasures: the baseball he'd gotten at his first Red Sox game (a foul ball caught by the man sitting in front of him), a replica of an 18th century Navy galleon Chris brought back for him after teaching one summer in Australia, a smooth stone plucked from the sandy beach on Prince Edward Island where we vacationed every summer, and ticket stubs and programs from games he'd attended. For Christmas the year before, we'd given him a specialized baseball bat he'd been coveting, and for weeks he slept with it tucked next to him in bed.

The new fishing rod ranked in the same value category. I gently took it out of his hands and examined the snarled line jamming the reel. It was wound pretty tightly, but I'd fished a lot with my father and brothers as a kid, and I had plenty of experience with these kinds of snares. "Hand me the scissors," I said. When he did, I cut into the bird's nest of crossed line to loosen the knots coiled near the spool. I wiggled the handle back and forth and cut another loop. The reel mechanism released and spun backwards, spitting out the rest of the jumbled fishing line. "There," I said, snipping the remaining knots off the spool and pulling out a single thread. "It's not broken. You just need to restring the rod." The whole process took me less than two minutes.

Will's shoulders released some of their stress, and he reached for the rod while he wiped his dripping nose on the sleeve of his gray t-shirt. Relief worked its way across his features "I've been trying to untangle it for the last forty-five minutes," he managed to say in between shuddering breaths.

My heart lurched. A mirror to Chris's personality, Will was my even-keeled child. He took things in stride, and rarely overreacted. I'd never seen him this upset, and picturing him sitting alone for that much time, agonizing over something so simple while working himself into this frenzy of worry made me want to cry. "Why didn't you call me?" I asked, my voice cracking on the final syllable.

"I sort of panicked, and I didn't want to bother you."

Will's words tugged at a particular loop in the snarl of my own adolescent memories that I'd been working to untangle. After my dad's diagnosis, I never wanted to bother my parents with my worry, either. They tried to hide the anxiety they felt, but its frightening presence was always there, weighing down the surrounding air. How could I add to that heaviness? I'd always thought. I didn't remember them ever doing or saying anything that told me I couldn't talk to them about what I was feeling, but I also knew they hadn't ever extended an explicit invitation that told me I could. That silence created a border I'd never dared to cross.

I did not want that border to exist for my children.

Ever.

I wrapped Will into a tight hug and held him close for a few seconds. He didn't pull away and leaned into the embrace. I breathed in the musty scent of his hair and felt the broad stretch of his back. He was not a little boy anymore. But he was nowhere close to being a grown up.

I pulled back, keeping my hands resting lightly on his shoulders for another moment and looked into his wet eyes. "You can always talk to me about how you are feeling," I said. "Always. You are never bothering me."

His eyes dropped, and a sheepish grin played on his lips. "I guess I just panicked," he said again, notes of apology and embarrassment filtering into the statement.

"I know what that feels like. It's the worst feeling in the world."

He looked up, his eyebrows a question.

"I don't want you to ever have to feel like that by yourself," I said. "You don't ever have to try to deal with things on your own." I rested my back against his bed and gestured at the fishing rod. "I know that this didn't turn out to be such a big deal. It was a pretty easy fix. But, as you get older, I'm sure there will be things that happen that might make you feel like this again. And maybe they won't be so easy to fix."

I wanted to make sure I got this next part right.

"You can always, *always* ask me or Dad for help. Even if it's something you're afraid might upset us or that we'll be mad about." I tossed out a few generic examples: getting stuck at a party where people were drinking or finding himself in a situation where his friends were doing things he didn't want to do. He was listening and storing my words in that quiet way of his. "No matter what it is, we will always take care of you first."

He fiddled with the loosened fishing line and threaded it into the metal guides up the length of the rod.

"Okay?" I asked.

"Okay."

He was back to himself, his breathing steady, his body relaxed. A calm settled around us, and we sat quietly for a couple of minutes. He finished stringing the rod, and then we both stood. I had to go get Lily. He had to return to his desk and the unfinished homework.

I leaned on his doorframe and watched Will open his algebra book and rip a lined sheet of paper from his notebook. His hand grasped the pencil firmly, and his forehead wrinkled in concentration as he worked out an equation on the page.

I could still see the tiny baby him. The tiny baby who'd arrived six weeks early and weighed just over four pounds. So fragile and defenseless. Was that who I'd always see? No matter how big he got? I felt the pull of longing. I wanted to keep all of life's hurt as far away as possible, but I couldn't.

My parents couldn't either. The secret that was meant to shelter us from the stain of HIV/AIDS didn't stop it from bleeding into our lives anyway. And maybe if I'd talked to them about it, if I'd felt like I could ask for help, I wouldn't have been so scared all the time.

I turned to leave but paused to look back at Will's bent head one more time.

"I love you," I said, trying to infuse the three familiar words with all the vital messages I wanted him to hear and internalize.

He glanced up from his work, his pencil suspended above the paper. "I know, Mom." There was confidence in his statement. Certainty painted his face. "I love you too."

He went back to his math, and I walked into the hallway, tucking his confidence close, understanding that though there was plenty I'd gotten wrong, in that moment, I was getting this part right. My feet sank into the soft carpet, and my eyes worked to adjust to the dark. In a few seconds, the shadows gave way, and I could make out my path to the stairs. Cautiously, I moved forward.

Epilogue
2014

THERE DAD WAS.

His tilted face filled the television's flat screen, captured by the camera's lens at extremely close range and cropped midway down his forehead, right above the permanent crease that dented the skin between his brows, and just below his disarming smile. His brown eyes, so alive with warmth and wisdom, crinkled behind the wired, rectangle frames of his eyeglasses. He was looking right at me.

But he wasn't. Dad's penetrating gaze was suspended in some unknown, distant interval of time. Somewhere out of my reach. The awareness of that expanse filled me with the same emptiness as always. I wanted to cry, but I clamped down on my back teeth and blinked over and over again, urging the tears to stay put. A nearly twenty-year-old question circled my brain: how could the man in this photo be dead?

"Aw, what a great picture," my sister-in-law, Ellen, said from her spot behind me where she'd pulled up one of the spindle-backed kitchen chairs.

It was night two of our annual Messenger family vacation on Prince Edward Island, and sixteen of us—nine adults and seven kids ranging in age from seventeen to nine—crowded into the tight living room space of Mark and Ellen's rented cottage. I was crammed on a plaid, upholstered couch with David and Mark. The fabric scratched against my bare legs. Mom sat in a cushioned chair across from me, and my brother-in-law, Ian, leaned against its arm, holding his phone that also served as the baby monitor for Ben, my sixteen-month-old nephew, asleep in their adjacent cottage. Chris and Yvonne had opted for kitchen chairs too. The rest of the kids lounged against each other or the furniture on the faux-wood laminate floor.

Wood was the defining décor of these rental cottages—specifically, pine. The knotty, paneled walls and high, sloping ceilings, the dining tables and chairs, the coffee and end tables, the kitchen cabinets, bed frames and bureaus. All pine. I might have opted for some color variety if I'd been charged with the interior design, but the cottages were clean and comfortable, and they provided a perfect location for my scattered family to gather for this one week every August.

"We're starting with shots of just Mom and Dad, some individual, some together," Michael said from his seat on the bottom of the stairs next to the TV. His MacBook rested on his knees and a thin cable stretched from it to the back of the television. After some technical wrangling that only he could accomplish, he'd figured out a way to stream these photos from his computer onto the larger screen, and, by default, was now the designated master of ceremonies for the proceedings.

He clicked to the next photo. This one showed a much younger version of Dad. He was pulling his snow-speckled overcoat close to his neck. His dark hair was dusted with snow, too, and from behind different glasses, smaller ones with black, plastic frames, ones considered vintage these days, he squinted into the camera against what appeared to be pelting snowflakes that swirled in the air around him. He was smiling, but this time it looked forced, almost pained, like he couldn't wait for the picture taking to be over. He stood against the backdrop of a rocky, snow-covered slope that led to a forest of leafless trees, their bare limbs etched with a thin layer of snow as well. In the far-left corner of the shot, the blurred edge of a car window said the photographer was sheltered inside the vehicle.

"I tried to divide the slides into categories: early pictures of Dad and me, then each of you as babies, then pictures of the whole family," Mom said. "But I didn't have time to put them in any order after that, so they aren't chronological. I don't know where or when that is," she added about the picture now on the screen.

"Nobody cares, Mom," Mark said. "It's just great to see them."

Mom's shoulders loosened, and she shifted to a more comfortable position in the chair, cradling a throw pillow in the crook of her arm.

Mom was divorcing John. She had decided in January. The split unfolded in a series of impulsive moves on her part that probably made things more painful than they needed to be for them both, but we were all relieved that she'd finally made the break. She'd wasted a lot of time trying to convince us (and herself) otherwise, but we knew how unhappy she was in her marriage to John. We weren't missing him. His presence in our family was never easy for him or for us to navigate, making for a lot of awkward interaction, at best. Though she had a lot of adjustment ahead of her, Mom seemed better. Lighter, somehow.

John had moved out of their condo at the beginning of June. Since his departure, Mom had been in a bit of an arranging/clearing-out/redis-covering her stuff, and herself, frenzy. Organizing things had always been a cathartic way for Mom to order life. As part of this most recent initiative, she'd cleared out a storage unit she'd been renting, obses-sively distributing to each of us pieces of furniture and sentimental items from her old home that she didn't have space for in her condo. My grandfather Messenger's wooden WWII trunk, carted down on a visit to us in May, now resided in Will's bedroom. Mom also rediscov-ered the boxes of family slides and spent the weeks before this vacation sorting through them. She selected about six hundred and got them put onto a CD. Since our arrival on the island, she'd been fixated on finding a time for us all to see them.

I sensed that there was a reordering happening here too. A deliberate effort to turn the camera away from the turbulence in her marriage to John and refocus the family lens on her life with Dad. An effort to recapture the person she was before this second marriage made her feel like she was supposed to sever the intimacies of those ties to Dad to allow room for a new husband.

I wasn't quite ready to trust it yet. This latest transition in what had been a parade of transition points for Mom since Dad died had unfurled some emotions inside me that weren't quite ready to be ordered.

But as Michael clicked through more of these opening snapshots, I welcomed the first chance in eight years to shine the spotlight fully on Dad, on Dad and Mom, on our family history, without having to tiptoe around anyone's feelings.

"Oh, wow," I breathed, when another photo of Dad, in his early twenties at most, flashed on the screen. It was a stunningly composed portrait. He sat sideways in the bow of an aluminum rowboat wearing a button-down, rusted plaid shirt and khaki pants. His elbows rested on his bent knees, and his thoughtful gaze was trained on the open page of the thin, weathered Bible he held in his hands. A lake stretched behind him, just out of focus, its perimeter lined with the blurred shapes of trees.

"That's in the Poconos," Mom said. "Our honeymoon."

Dad was twenty-three then. A month out of medical school and at the start of his adult life. The same age I was when he died. This was the entry point for our family. Pure. That was the descriptor that jumped into my head. It all looked so untainted.

What was he reading? What scriptural promise was shaping this moment for him? For my mother, too, the photographer at the other end of the rowboat?

Scattered among the more familiar images of Mom and Dad in this first collection, images of times I'd witnessed or photos I remembered seeing before, were more of these honeymoon shots. Breathtaking and optimistic reflections of my parents at the dawn of their life together. There was a gorgeous one of Mom caught mid-flight on a chain swing, about to soar off the screen. Her fashionably bobbed hair wisped against her cheek and even from this side-view, her bright, wistful smile was visible. In this carefree and unstaged instant, she was beautiful.

I wanted this photograph on my wall at home. This one and the one of Dad in the rowboat. I wanted them even though they delivered a host of complicated feelings: Joy. Sadness. Awe. Longing. I wanted to hold the memories of these moments, even though I knew the crushing reality of what came later.

"Grandma, you are so pretty," my niece Rose declared.

"That was a long time ago," Mom said.

My mother was still beautiful. Her smooth skin, regal features, and deep blue eyes made her appear younger than her seventy-one years. When she stopped coloring her hair a few years ago and cropped it into an edgy, no-fuss style, people consistently started comparing her to the actress Helen Mirren.

None of the grandkids had ever seen any early images like these. The story unfolding in this mishmash of pictures was one they didn't know, I realized. It was hard for me to keep from blaming Mom and her marriage to John for this disconnect, to keep from making her the culprit in this narrative gap. But it was not just Mom. It was me. It was all of us. Even Dad. Silence was our family history.

The slideshow continued, and in a slew of individual close-ups of chubby cheeks and gummy smiles, Michael, Mark, David, and I broke onto the scene. Extended choruses of "aw" and "look how cute" came from the kids as a series of photos of each of us in various stages of baby and toddlerhood cycled across the screen.

"Oh my word!" Mom exclaimed, leaning forward in her seat, when a picture of Michael came up. He was about eighteen months old, staring thoughtfully into the camera. "That looks so much like Ben!"

She was right. There was something in the shape of the eyes, the curve of the lips, the contour of the chin that resembled my little nephew, more so than David's baby pictures, even. Family genes had flowed through the new generation of Messengers in unexpected ways. I looked over at Will, who reclined back on his elbows next to Rose in front of my mother's chair. Their heads tilted in the same way as they scrutinized the photos on the screen. They were almost exactly a year apart, and with their strawberry-tinted hair, their freckled noses, and rounded cheeks, they looked more like brother and sister than Will and Lily did. "Twinsies" we'd jokingly called them since they were little. Not only did they look alike, but with their dry humor and their general lack of self-consciousness, they acted alike too.

When my oldest niece, Madeline, was born just a year after Dad died, I couldn't stop seeing his expressions all over her face. He never had the chance to meet any of his eight grandchildren, but in striking ways, Dad had managed to show up in each one of them.

After the baby photos came the family shots. A chain of captured memories meandering through Christmases, camping expeditions, ski vacations, road trips, summers spent at our cottage on Main River in Kent County, New Brunswick.

The unfortunate styles of the late seventies and eighties in these photographs roused a lot of laughter and a flurry of sarcastic comments from the kids.

"Nice socks, Uncle Mike," Madeline teased about a photo of Michael in his mid-teens, clad in short shorts and calf-length tube socks.

"Nice legs too," my nephew Aidan added.

"Um, Mom, what exactly is going on with your hair?" Lily asked as one bad perm followed another through my early adolescence and teen years.

"Uncle Mark, you look exactly the same," Will commented. It was true. We often joked that Mark's face and hair had not undergone any dramatic variations since he was a teenager. You could line up his high school, college, medical school, and wedding photos and only be able to identify the era by what he was wearing.

"Is that PEI?" David asked when the next picture appeared. Mom, Michael, Mark, and I sat together on a blanket, a collection of shovels, pails, coolers, and beach chairs strewn around us. David, his naked toddler body wrapped only in a sagging, white beach towel, appeared to be on the run across the red sand. Ocean waves lapped against the shore in the background, the water and cloudless sky reflecting the same cerulean blue.

"I think that's Cavendish," Mom said.

Cavendish was the beach a mile down the road from these cottages. The beach where we spent the bulk of our days on this yearly vacation. Where we'd sat this afternoon and watched the kids dodge this year's influx of jellyfish in the surf.

In the next image, David sat in the wet sand at the beach's waterline, playing with a green plastic boat. Dad, shirtless, tanned, and healthy, squatted beside him, his eyes hidden behind dark sunglasses, a relaxed smile stretching across his face.

For an instant, the tow-headed, toddler version of David morphed into Will at that age, and I glimpsed my dad with my son, playing in the same sand. A picture I yearned for all the time. A picture I'd never have.

I dug my fingers into the couch cushion, my heart pounding, and let my eyes drift around the room, trying to read the expressions of my brothers and mother. I could see on their faces the private workings of their own brains as they came face-to-face with the images of a life that had vanished.

I wanted to talk about it. I wanted to know if my brothers and mother felt the same gaping emptiness that I did when they looked at these pictures of Dad on the same beach where we'd vacationed without him for thirteen years. The pictures that we could arrange and rearrange but would still spell out the same ending—Dad's absence.

I wasn't brave enough to start the conversation, though. I never was. If nobody else was talking about it, maybe I shouldn't, either. I didn't want to be the perceived downer in the room. A photo of Michael, Mark, and me a couple of years before David was born had caught my attention earlier. It seemed to say something about the way things worked in our family. I was about three, so Mark would be five and Michael six. In a comic portrayal of the sibling hierarchy, Michael was seated on a gold-painted, raised throne at some amusement park, and Mark and I flanked him on either side sitting on low, folding stools. Michael stared straight into the camera, smug satisfaction defining his smile. Mark seemed to have caught sight of something entertaining beyond the photographer, and his lips played into a sly grin. But I was not looking in either of the directions that they were. My hands held my bare knees to my chest, and my face turned to the side, my eyes squinting toward my brothers, watching them.

Things hadn't changed a whole lot since then.

I met Chris's eyes for a minute. His brow furrowed, his head tilted just a little like he was about to ask a question, I knew he sensed some of my internal struggle. I looked away. My sadness was ratcheted up by the last few weeks of my writing about the agonizing final days of Dad's life. Scenes I'd have to revisit later tonight because my deadline for these latest chapters of my MFA thesis was the next day. Writing had stirred up different snapshots than the ones we'd just seen. Snapshots no one wanted to linger over, and the hardest pages yet. But I didn't talk about those pages now. I didn't talk about any of it because I was starting to understand that the way I felt things didn't have to be the way the rest of my family felt things for my feelings to be okay.

We continued to reminisce about family trips and holidays as the final set of photos captured us in various groupings and poses next to recognizable landmarks: a ski hill in Vermont, a lighthouse in New Brunswick, a sign at the entrance to Disney World. "That was great, Mom," Michael said as the last one—a snapshot of us all except Mark (the likely photographer) standing in front of Buckingham Palace from our trip to England only months before Dad's heart attack—faded from the screen. He unhooked his laptop from the television, pushing the off button on the TV.

"It was," everyone else chimed in, stretching and getting up from spots around the room.

"I'm sorry about some of the mistakes," Mom apologized, the same flutter of worry making her voice breathless. In a few places, she'd mixed up some of our baby photos and inadvertently inserted a few strangers into the midst of the family shots. Among some of the favorite pictures of Dad fly fishing on rivers in New Brunswick had been a gorgeous photo featuring a man none of us, including Mom, could identify.

We reassured her again that we were just happy to have the memories. That it wasn't about the order. Or things being perfect.

"Anyone want coffee?" Ellen offered, and dragged the kitchen chairs back to the table. There were no takers. Dave and Ian bowed out and headed back to their cottage to check on Ben.

"I'm beat," Mom said mid-yawn and got to her feet. "I think I'm going to say goodnight too." She followed the guys out the door. Relief had softened the lines in her forehead, and I could almost picture the X marking a box on her never-ending mental to-do list: slideshow viewing, done.

Mike folded his laptop, and with some parting words about a potential deep-sea fishing expedition the next day, he and Yvonne disappeared out the door too.

The kids had already scattered in different directions with various electronic devices, and Chris and Will, hoping to catch some of the Red Sox game, returned to our cottage.

Now that Dave and I had vacated it, Mark was reclined on the couch, his bare feet stretching past the end, a pillow propped under his head. His eyes were already drooping toward sleep.

I'd expected something. Something comforting as, together, we caught a glimpse of a family that once was. Instead, I felt the swell of sadness inside me begin to deflate. Maybe there didn't need to be anything else. Maybe my expectations were set a little too high.

"Thanks for hosting," I smiled to Ellen and made my way to the door.

"'Night, Melster," Mark said lazily from the couch.

—

No one had bothered to turn on the outside lights, and the dim glow from the shaded cottage windows did little to disperse the darkness around me when I stepped out into the night. The air was dewy and warm against my skin. The gravel crunched under my flip flops as I followed the path to our cottage. I stopped halfway across the space between the two buildings and tilted my head back to look at the stretch of sky overhead. Something about the island geography, the nearness of the ocean, made the sky feel bigger here. Stars punctured the black, tiny pinpricks of light shaping into familiar constellations.

"Here, I'll help you trace it," Dad's voice echoed somewhere deep in the recesses of my brain and a memory sharpened. We were sprawled side by side on a thick, shag carpet in the family room of our summer cottage in New Brunswick. The lights were off so we could stare out at the night sky through the panoramic window that took up most of the front wall and showcased the view of the river. On this night when I was about nine, it was so clear we could see satellites tracking paths among the brilliant sea of stars. While Mom and David searched for signs of the anticipated meteor shower, Michael and Mark had been pointing out the different constellations, competing to see who could spot them first.

"I see Orion," Mark declared with triumph.

"I found that five minutes ago," Michael said.

I was still trying to locate the Big Dipper.

Dad closed his hand over mine and pointed my finger to a particularly bright star. "That's the North Star," he said. "Always look for that one first. It helps you to clear the clutter of all the other ones." He moved my finger in a straight line from that star to another bright one a few inches below it. "Now this is the edge of the Big Dipper," he said. "It's made up of these seven bright stars." He drew a shape with my finger. "Think of a big soup ladle, or even the shape of a wheelbarrow," he said.

I focused my eyes on those stars as he traced the shape again. And, just like that, I saw it. "There!" I cried, triumphant satisfaction and wonder mingling in a single word.

"There," Dad said, and drew my finger back up to the North Star. "Now, see if you can find the Little Dipper too. The North Star is at the tip of its handle."

I found it right away. Dad released his grip on my hand, and I rested my head against his shoulder and stared up at the Big Dipper and the Little Dipper, tracing their lines with my finger over and over again. The two constellations stood out from all of the other stars. I felt like I'd been let in on an important secret.

"From now on, you'll always know how to find them without anybody's help," Dad said.

More than thirty years later, the same starry canvas gazed down on me where I stood between the cottages and I couldn't help feeling that infinite space cluttered with so many of my habitual questions always too big for answers. Why didn't the boys and Mom linger in their grief the way I did when confronted with images of what could have been? Why weren't the words of regret and loss and longing I so wanted to speak the same words that rested on their tongues? Why were they so quick to shut down moments like tonight that opened up space to remember? As the disappointment of yet another gathering of unrealized expectations tried to take hold, a concession funneled into my mind. I couldn't know what was inside of them any more than they could know what was inside of me. A fresh question surfaced. Why did their responses matter so much? And that night, for the first time, I considered a new answer.

Maybe they didn't.

It felt like opening a release valve on a pressurized tank. All the pent-up frustrations leaking out in one, swift whoosh, leaving room for an emerging, gentler clarity.

It didn't matter whether my search was their search. What mattered was that my search was leading me toward something that I was starting to recognize as important and necessary even though I could not yet see the constellation for the stars.

I could not yet see that reaching back and tracing the history that landed my family where it did would be my path forward. That I would eventually choose to let go and leave behind some of the questions that weren't really mine to answer.

That naming all the things I couldn't say for all those years would expand the isolated narrative of our story—the official version I'd tried so hard, but failed, to navigate—in beautiful and unexpected ways. That it would allow me the privilege of meeting and learning from other people who'd courageously written their tough stories, people who would become trusted companions along the way and extend to me generous words of encouragement and wisdom that would fill the pages of my first published book, *Writing Hard Stories: Celebrated Memoirists Who Shaped Art from Trauma*. That one of those memoirists would introduce me to an entire community of children of my generation who'd lost parents to AIDS, *The Recollectors*, and encourage me to write an essay for them to publish. And that on a cold December night in 2015, I would stand in a packed room at a World AIDS Day event in New York City and read that essay—now a chapter in this story—to a group of strangers who, because of the common threads of our experiences, wouldn't be strangers after all.

That I would continue to share pieces of this story and interrogate where it began, publishing more essays on topics of illness, grief, and justice. That I would be emboldened to speak in front of more people, understanding that in doing so, I would open space for them to lean into my experiences and find courage to reveal some of their own.

That in the intimate spaces with Chris and Will and Lily, I would shed past family definitions of perceived resilience on which I'd hinged my identity, and make room for what existed beneath—a more authentic me who recognized the strength in being vulnerable with each other.

I could not yet see that I would even take cautious steps back toward my Christian faith, honoring my need to understand how the roots of the church and my family and my father wound into the roots of me. That one Sunday Chris and I would visit a church only blocks from our home that we'd passed thousands of times, but never entered, sit in the pew and listen to the gentle-voiced minister begin the service with the words, "No matter who you are, whom you love, or where you are on life's journey, you are welcome here," and that instead of wanting to flee, I would feel a pull to stay.

I could not yet see that at the very moment I'd be ready to publish this book, a new pandemic would rage across the globe, impacting us all, and carrying with it haunting reverberations of the early AIDS crisis. That twenty-five years after my father's death, his story and the stories of countless other victims of HIV/AIDS would hold lessons for our present crisis and continue to resonate.

But that August night, I couldn't see any of these things. What I could see was the North Star, still and sure at the center of the sky. A fixed point. A beacon. In various cultures across the world, the Big Dipper is part of the cultural mythology. In Greek stories, it's known as the Great Bear. In Ireland and the UK, the Plough. In Germany, it's called the Great Cart, and in Italy, the Great Wagon. However, in an old Arabic legend, the four stars that make up the asterism's bowl symbolize a coffin, and the three stars of the handle are the mourners who follow after the deceased.

I stretched my finger and followed an ascending path to the star representing the final mourner at the tip of the Big Dipper.

"There," I said softly and dropped my hand to my side. The sound of my voice drifted on the air and trailed upward, expectant. Limitless.

Acknowledgements

Many people have accompanied me on the writing path that has stretched ten years from this book's beginnings to its publication, and I am grateful for the opportunity to say thank you.

I'm indebted to Jessica Bell, Amie McCracken, and the amazing team at Vine Leaves Press for publishing *A Hard Silence*, and to Alexis Paige, my VLP developmental editor and generous friend, for believing in this story, taking such good care of it along the way, and helping me get it just right.

My appreciation to the editors of the following publications in which pieces of this book originally appeared: *Modern Loss, Bustle, Word Riot,* and *The Recollectors.*

Thank you to my faculty mentors in the Stonecoast MFA program whose support and guidance helped me to shape early pieces of this narrative, and whose friendships have anchored me in the years since. Jaed Coffin urged me to generate and generate some more, giving me permission to stop worrying about shape and structure. Susan Conley gently prodded me toward the scenes that are at the heart of this story and taught me to linger there long enough to figure out what I really needed to say. And Suzanne Strempek Shea, who read multiple drafts of this narrative, who comforted me through weepy phone calls when it all felt too hard, who shared an endless supply of resources, who never faltered in her belief that this book would find its way into the world even when I was ready to give up, is a life gift for whom I will never have enough thank yous.

Special appreciation goes to the eighteen authors who spoke to me for my first book, *Writing Hard Stories: Celebrated Memoirists Who*

Shaped Art from Trauma (Beacon Press), and whose shared wisdom about their own writing journeys gave me the necessary grounding to continue with mine: Andre Dubus III, Sue William Silverman, Michael Patrick McDonald, Joan Wickersham, Kyoko Mori, Richard Hoffman, Suzanne Strempek Shea, Abigail Thomas, Monica Wood, Mark Doty, Edwidge Danticat, Marianne Leone, Jerald Walker, Kate Bornstein, Jessica Handler, Richard Blanco, Alysia Abbott, and Kim Stafford.

I'm deeply grateful to my amazing friends who are also writers and who understand just what it means to do this work, so many of whom, at different times, have read iterations of this story and offered feedback or simply given their encouragement: Jennifer Dupree, Danara Wallace, Elisha Emerson, Penny Guisinger, Amanda Silva, Betsy Small Campbell, Jess Pulver, Anne Pinkerton, Yi Shun Lai, Julia Munemo, Lynn Hall, Dana Mich, Lisa Cooper Ellison, Tommy Shea, and Sonia Ascher.

So much gratitude to my beautiful and talented friend Gretchen Warsen who is not a writer, but a painter, and talks me off the precipice multiple times a day because she knows the challenges of balancing a creative life with just life.

I'm also deeply grateful to have a loyal community of caring friends who regularly pull me away from the isolation of my writing chair for long walks, coffee dates, lengthy phone calls, cookie decorating sessions, and pickle ball games: Meg Gould, Hillari Wennerstrom, Shayna Burgher, Sherri Renwick, Julie Norris, Maureen Curran, Penny Jamerson, Katie Kramarczyk, and Madeleine Dockrill.

Sincere thanks to Dr. B, my first reader, long before there were even pages to read: it's impossible to express how vital the trusted space of his office has been to this creative (and often painful) process.

Love and gratitude to my mother and three brothers, who've lived their own stories of this story, for their support throughout this process, despite the painful wounds that it understandably opens for them.

Endless adoration for my children, Will and Lily, who rallied when I dropped the parenting ball, when I was absent, when the stress spilled over. They have become incredible adults who appreciate their mother, scars and all. They are the reasons I needed to unpack this story and learn to carry it differently.

Finally and always, to Chris: Thanks to him for holding our family together, for sacrificing so much, for complaining so little. For traveling this life with me. He is my safest of spaces, my biggest support, my best and favorite friend.

Vine Leaves Press

Enjoyed this book?
Go to *vineleavespress.com* to find more.
Subscribe to our newsletter:

CPSIA information can be obtained
at www.ICGtesting.com
Printed in the USA
JSHW030733210623
43527JS00006B/26